UNDERSTANDING WOUNDS

A NURSE'S GUIDE

BY
DR. SANDRA WITHERS

TABLE OF CONTENTS

ABOUT THE AUTHOR

Dr. Sandra Withers, PhD, MSN, BSN, RN, Director of Nursing | Clinical Educator Dr. Sandra Withers is a dedicated healthcare leader, educator, and clinician with over 30 years of experience in nursing and patient care. As a Registered Nurse holding a Bachelor of Science in Nursing (BSN) and a Master of Science in Nursing (MSN), Dr. Withers has built her career around a strong foundation of clinical excellence, with a special focus on wound care and management. Her PhD in Psychology further enhances her approach, allowing her to see patient care through both physical and emotional lenses.

Throughout her career, Dr. Withers has served in a range of healthcare settings, from hospitals to home health, rising to the role of Director of Nursing. In this capacity, she has led clinical teams, developed training programs, and launched quality initiatives aimed at improving patient outcomes. Her passion for wound care comes from her mission to give nurses and clinicians the knowledge and hands-on skills they need to manage complex wounds with confidence.

Dr. Withers is equally committed to advancing nursing education and professional growth. She has mentored countless nurses, helping them build the competence and self-assurance essential for excellent clinical practice. Her combined expertise in nursing and psychology shapes her holistic philosophy of care, which prioritizes both effective treatment and compassionate support for patients' overall well-being.

With Understanding Wounds: A Nurse's Guide, Dr. Withers shares decades of practical insight in an accessible resource designed for nurses, students, and healthcare professionals. This guide reflects her lifelong commitment to raising wound care standards, improving clinical results, and empowering providers to deliver patient-centered, evidence-based care. Driven by her belief that every nurse deserves the right tools to thrive and that every patient deserves the highest standard of care, Dr. Withers continues to champion excellence in nursing practice.

DEDICATION

This guide is dedicated to God—our ultimate source of wisdom and healing and my awesome family. It is by divine grace that we are equipped with the knowledge, discernment, and compassion to provide care that restores not just the body, but the dignity of every patient. May this book serve as a practical resource and a reminder of the sacred responsibility we carry as nurses in promoting evidence-based healing and safety.

ABOUT THE BOOK

Understanding Wounds: A Nurse's Guide is an essential resource tailored specifically for nurses, particularly those practicing in Home Health. In this setting, nurses often work independently, with limited immediate clinical support, making sound wound care knowledge not just valuable—but necessary.

This guide provides practical, easy-to-understand information while maintaining clinical depth. It covers wound types, proper assessment, measurement techniques, documentation standards, and evidence-based interventions that align with industry guidelines, including WOCN standards. Whether managing surgical wounds, pressure injuries, diabetic ulcers, Arterial wounds, venous stasis wounds or complex non-healing wounds, nurses will find concise, actionable insights to improve patient outcomes.

Designed for quick reference in the field, this book empowers nurses to deliver high-quality care confidently and competently. Although easy to read, each page is packed with vital knowledge that can transform practice, enhance critical thinking, and strengthen clinical decision-making in wound management.

For the Home Health nurse, Understanding Wounds is not just a book—it is a reliable companion for safe, effective, and informed wound care.

INTRODUCTION

Wound management is a critical component of nursing care across all healthcare settings. As wounds grow increasingly complex due to chronic conditions, surgical interventions, and aging populations, clinicians must be equipped with up-to-date knowledge, practical skills, and sound clinical judgment to assess, manage, and promote wound healing effectively.

Understanding Wounds: A Nurse's Guide was developed to provide a clear, accessible, and evidence-based resource rooted in best practices, including guidelines from the Wound, Ostomy, and Continence Nurses Society (WOCN®).

This guide addresses the fundamental principles of wound assessment, classification, documentation, and treatment. It also highlights appropriate use of wound care products, advanced therapies, and decision-making pathways in managing wound types, including pressure injuries, surgical wounds, and diabetic foot ulcers.

It is intended for nurses at all levels—students, bedside clinicians, field clinicians, and wound care specialists—as a reliable reference in the pursuit of excellence in wound care. Family caregivers and interdisciplinary team members may also find this resource valuable in understanding their role in supporting wound healing and preventing complications.

May this guide enhance your clinical confidence, reinforce critical thinking, and ultimately improve the quality of care delivered to every patient. The goal is not only to treat wounds but to promote healing, prevent recurrence, and restore dignity and quality of life to those we serve.

CHAPTER 1
Understanding the Spectrum of Wounds

Each chapter of this book will equip the nurse with a renewed clarity of the fundamentals of wound care, while empowering caregivers and families to recognize and respond to wounds with confidence and urgency. Wound care is both a science and an art — a careful balancing act of assessment, observation, and intervention. For the nurse at the bedside, the subtle changes in skin color, temperature, and sensation can be the earliest signs of something much deeper developing beneath the surface. For the patient or caregiver, those same signs may be easy to overlook until they become painful or complicated.

Understanding Wounds: A Nurse's Guide will walk you through the major categories of pressure-related wounds, stage by stage, beginning with the most subtle changes in skin integrity and progressing to the most severe tissue destruction. It will also explore other types of wounds, such as arterial wounds, venous wounds, diabetic wounds, and surgical wounds, highlighting the unique characteristics and care considerations of each. Whether you are a nurse in the field, or a student beginning your journey into wound care, or a family member learning to support a loved one, understanding these stages is crucial to early detection, timely intervention, and optimal healing.

Each chapter will begin with plain-language descriptions — such as "The skin is red, but not broken," designed to help non-clinicians grasp what they are seeing. Then, I will delve deeper into the clinical indicators: What makes a Stage 1 wound different from a Stage 2? What signs signal the need for urgent debridement? Why might a patient with a Stage 4 wound feel little to no pain at the wound center?

Alongside each clinical explanation, you will find visual aids, case examples, and caregiver tips, in addition to symptom insights and real-world cues that make wounds easier to recognize in both home and clinical settings.

Pressure Ulcers

Pressure ulcers, also known as pressure injuries or bedsores, are localized areas of tissue damage caused by prolonged pressure, shear, or friction. A unique and critical aspect of pressure ulcers is that they are stageable. Unlike many other wounds, pressure ulcers are categorized into specific stages that reflect the depth and severity of tissue involvement—from Stage 1, where the skin is intact but shows early signs of injury, to Stage 4, where deeper structures such as muscle, tendon, or bone are exposed.

This staging system provides a standardized framework for assessment, documentation, and treatment planning. It allows healthcare professionals to clearly identify the progression of tissue damage, implement timely interventions, and evaluate healing outcomes. Understanding that pressure ulcers are stageable emphasizes the importance of accurate wound assessment, as misclassification can lead to delays in care, inappropriate treatment, and compromised patient safety.

Consider the following stages of pressure Ulcers:

- **Stage 1**

Stage 1 pressure injury may seem like simple redness, but that persistent, non-blanchable erythema, often accompanied by warmth or pruritus.. At this stage, the skin is still intact, but the underlying tissue is already under stress. Early recognition and pressure relief can often reverse damage before it progresses.

- **Stage 2**

Stage 2 wounds mean the skin is broken. There may be a blister or shallow sore. Pain intensifies, and the wound bed appears moist and pink or red. Stage 2 is partial-thickness skin loss involving the epidermis and part of the dermis. Prompt protection of the wound bed and relief of pressure are critical to prevent advancement.

- **Stage 3**

Stage 3 wounds reveal yellow fat and tunneling beneath the surface, signaling full-thickness skin loss and the start of structural damage. The wound bed may contain granulation tissue, slough, or undermining. At this stage, infection risk is high, and specialized wound care, including possible debridement and advanced dressings becomes necessary.

- **Stage 4**

Stage 4 wounds are severe and critical. Bone, tendon, or muscle may be visible. The wound is deep, complex, and often accompanied by infection. Undermining and sinus tracts are common, and the healing process is prolonged. Stage 4 wounds are not only painful but also carry serious risks such as sepsis or osteomyelitis.

- **Unstageable**

Unstageable pressure injuries also fall into this category, where they are hidden behind layers of dead tissue, making visual assessment impossible without removal. Only after debridement can the true depth and severity be determined.

A Deep Tissue Pressure Injury (DTPI)

DTPI is a localized area of persistent, non-blanchable deep red, maroon, or purple discoloration of the skin, the skin may appear intact, but damage lurks below, revealing itself only when the skin collapses. This "bruise-like" appearance signals significant injury to the underlying soft tissue. DTPI is often caused by prolonged pressure or shear that damages tissue beneath intact skin because they can rapidly evolve into Stage 3 or Stage 4 wounds, DTPIs are sometimes called "silent threats." Early offloading and vigilant monitoring are crucial.

CHAPTER 2

Overview of Skin and Underlying Structures

The skin is the body's largest organ and its first line of defense, serving as both a protective barrier and a dynamic system that supports overall health. Structurally, the skin is composed of three primary layers—epidermis, dermis, and subcutaneous tissue (hypodermis)—each with a unique role in maintaining integrity, sensation, and healing.

The epidermis, the outermost layer, acts as a shield against pathogens, chemicals, and environmental stressors while regulating water loss.

Beneath it lies the dermis, a thicker layer rich in collagen, elastin, blood vessels, and nerves, which provides strength, flexibility, sensation, and thermoregulation.

The deepest layer, the subcutaneous tissue, is made up of fat and connective tissue that cushions internal structures, stores energy, and helps insulate the body.

Together, these layers form a coordinated system that protects, nourishes, and repairs itself. Understanding the anatomy of the skin is essential in wound care, as the depth of tissue involvement determines both the severity of the wound and the clinical approach required for healing.

1. Epidermis

The outermost layer of the skin. The epidermis is a thin, protective barrier composed primarily of keratinocytes. It is avascular (no blood vessels) and is nourished by the dermis below.

Functions:

- Protects against environmental hazards (bacteria, UV, water loss)
- Renews itself every 28–40 days through continuous cell turnover
- Regenerates quickly after superficial injuries
- In wound care, involvement is typically limited to minor abrasions and Stage 1 pressure injuries

Overview of the Skin and Underlying Structures

Epidermis

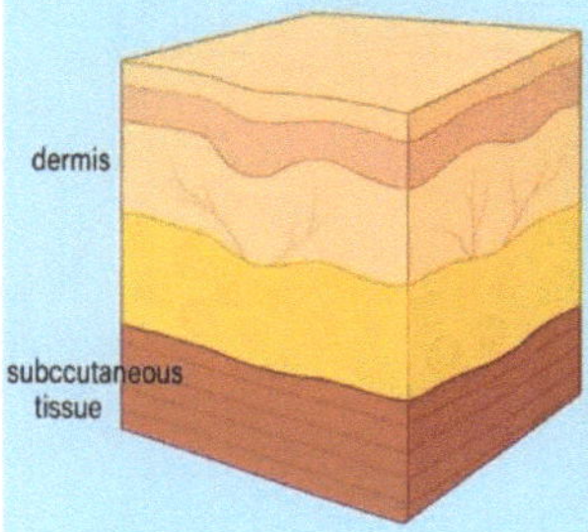

Outermost layer of the skin

The epidermis is a thin, protective barrier commosed primarily of keratinocytes. It is avascular (no blod vessels) and is nourished by dermis blo.

Functions:

- Protects against environmental hazards (bacteria, UV, water loss)
- Regenerate quiickly after superficial injuries

Damage includes minor abresions Stage 1 pressure injuries

2. Dermis

The dermis is the middle layer beneath the epidermis and is composed of collagen, elastin, nerve endings, blood vessels, and lymphatics. It contains the following:

- Hair follicles
- Sweat and sebaceous glands
- Capillaries and immune cells
- Fibroblasts, which produce collagen and play a vital role in wound healing
- Partial-thickness wounds extend into this layer
- Painful when exposed due to nerve endings

Overview of the Skin and Underlying Structures

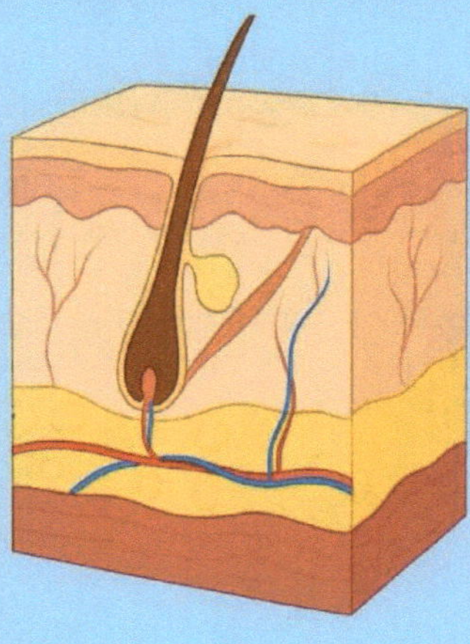

Dermis

The dermis is the middle layer beneath the epidermis and is composed of collagen, elastin, nerve endings, blood vessels, and lymphatics It contains the following:

- Hair follicles
- Sweat and sebaceous glands
- Capillaries and immune cells
- Partial-thickness wounds extend into this layer
- Painful when exposed due to nerve endings

3. Subcutaneous Tissue (Hypodermis)

The subcutaneous tissue is the layer of fat and connective tissue below the dermis.

Functions:

- Provides insulation, shock absorption, and energy storage
- Houses larger blood vessels and nerves
- Full-thickness wounds often extend into or through this layer
- Appears yellow and fatty in wounds
- Serves as a cushion protecting muscles and bones from external trauma

Subcutaneous Tissue (Hypodermis)

The subcutaneous tissue is layerof· fat and connective tissue below the dermis.

Functions:

- Provides insulation, shock absorption, and energy storage
- Houses larger blood vessels and nerves
- Full-thickness wounds often extend into this layer
- Appears ylowo and fatty in wounds

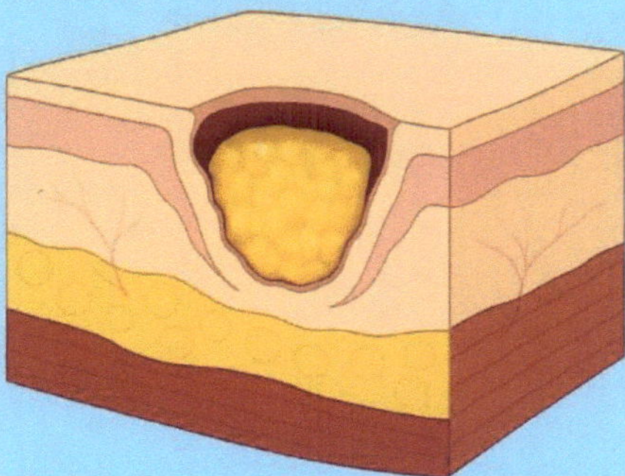

Beneath these layers are muscle and bone. While they are not considered part of the skin itself, they are important in wound care and pressure injury staging because severe wounds (Stage 4 pressure ulcers, for example) may extend through all layers of the skin and expose muscle or even bone.

Beneath these layers are muscle and bone. While they are not considered part of the skin itself, they are important in wound care and pressure injury staging because severe wounds (Stage 4 pressure ulcers, for example) may extend through all layers of the skin and expose muscle or even bone.

Muscle

The muscle lies beneath subcutaneous fat, it controls movement and posture. This area is highly vascularized, appears red, and striated. Exposure to the muscle indicates a Stage 4 pressure injury because of a rich blood supply, muscle tissue is prone to rapid necrosis if not perfused. Involvement of muscle increases infection risk and significantly delays wound healing injury.

Muscle

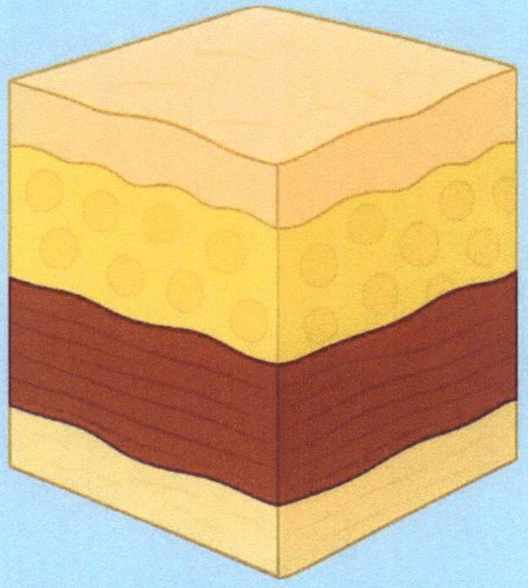

- Lies beneath subcutaneous fat, controls movament and posture
- Area is highly vascularized, appears red and striated
- Exposure to muscle indicates a Stage 4 pressure injury

Bone

The bone is the deepest structure affected by the most severe wounds. It supports and protects the body, serves as attachment for muscles. Exposure also indicates a Stage 4 pressure injury and carries high risk of osteomyelitis (bone infection).

Bone

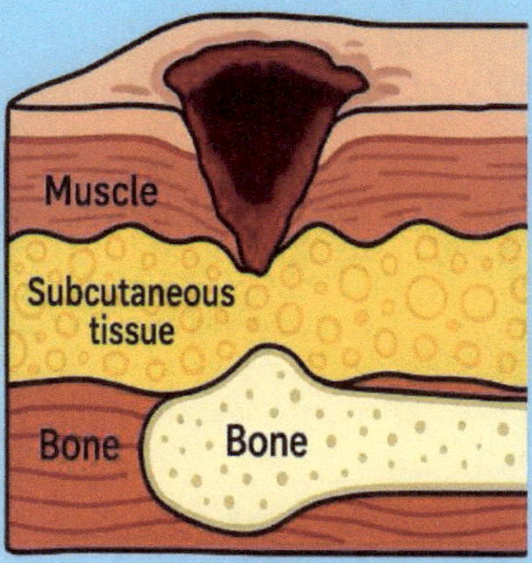

- Bone is the deepest structure affected by the most severe wounds
- Supports and protects the body, serves as attachment for muscles
- Exposure indicates Stage 4 pressure injury
- High risk of osteomyelitis (bone infection)

Summary Table

Layer	Key Characteristics	Seen in Wound Stage
Epidermis	Thin, outermost layer, no blood vessels	Stage 1
Dermis	Collagen-rich, vascular, nerve endings	Stage 2
Subcutaneous	Fatty, insulating layer	Stage 3
Muscle	Red, striated, vascular	Stage 4
Bone	Hard, deep structural tissue	Stage 4

CHAPTER 3

Pathophysiology of Pressure-Induced Tissue Damage

How Pressure Causes Tissue Damage

Pressure causes tissue damage by reducing or completely cutting off blood flow to the affected area. When pressure is sustained, especially over bony prominences, it compresses blood vessels and deprives tissues of oxygen and nutrients. This leads to cell death, inflammation, and eventually skin breakdown, beginning at the deepest layers and progressing outward.

Causes

1. Prolonged Pressure on Soft Tissue

When a patient lies or sits in one position for too long, external pressure exceeds capillary pressure (≈ 25–32 mmHg).

Common over bony prominences like sacrum, heels, hips, elbows, and occiput.

This compresses blood vessels, particularly the capillaries in the dermis and subcutaneous tissue.

2. Ischemia (Lack of Blood Flow)

Blood carries oxygen and nutrients vital for tissue survival.

Sustained pressure reduces or completely occludes blood flow to the area.

Without oxygen (hypoxia), cells begin to malfunction and die.

Tissues most sensitive to ischemia (e.g., muscle) are affected before the skin shows any signs.

3. Hypoxia → Metabolic Waste Accumulation

Impaired circulation also traps waste products and CO_2, causing:

- Acidosis
- Cellular edema
- Inflammation

4. Cellular Death and Necrosis

As ischemia continues (usually within 2 hours), cells begin to die.

Necrosis sets in:

- Erythema (redness) – initial tissue response
- Purplish/blue discoloration – deep tissue compromise
- Eschar (black, dry necrosis) or slough (yellow, devitalized tissue) in advanced stages
- Skin may remain intact even when deeper tissues are necrotic (as in DTPI).

5. Tissue Breakdown

Dead tissue triggers an inflammatory response, leading to:

- Enzymatic digestion of cells
- Invasion by bacteria
- Expansion of wound depth and infection risk

As the cascade continues, local tissue damage can spread, creating undermining and tunneling in advanced ulcers. This progression results in a visible wound, a pressure injury.

Summary of Key Mechanism

Stage	Event
Pressure	Sustained external force over tissue, especially near bony areas
Ischemia	Blocked blood flow, oxygen deprivation
Hypoxia	Cells starved of oxygen, energy failure begins
Necrosis	Tissue death from prolonged ischemia
Breakdown	Inflammatory enzymes and/or infection degrade tissue

Clinical Note

Factors such as shear, friction, and moisture can accelerate tissue breakdown by compounding ischemic damage. Importantly, muscle and adipose tissue may sustain severe injury before the skin shows visible signs, making early prevention strategies (e.g., repositioning, pressure redistribution devices) critical to patient safety.

CHAPTER 4
Understanding Wounds

What is a Wound?

A wound is defined as a disruption in the normal integrity of the skin and underlying tissues. The skin, being the body's first line of defense, protects against infection, regulates temperature, and prevents fluid loss. When that barrier is broken—whether by trauma, surgery, or underlying disease—healing becomes a complex process involving inflammation, tissue regeneration, and repair.

Wounds may range from superficial injuries such as abrasions to deep, complex wounds involving muscles, tendons, and even bone. They can be acute, chronic, open, or closed, and each requires a tailored approach to healing. Understanding the types of wounds and their unique characteristics is essential to providing proper care, promoting healing, and preventing complications.

Types of Wounds

1. Acute vs. Chronic Wounds

Acute Wounds: Result from sudden injury (such as cuts, abrasions, surgical incisions). They generally follow a predictable healing pattern.

Chronic Wounds: Fail to progress through normal healing stages, often due to poor circulation, infection, pressure, or underlying medical conditions. Examples include pressure injuries, venous ulcers, and diabetic ulcers.

2. Open vs. Closed Wounds

Open Wounds: Skin surface is broken, exposing tissue beneath (e.g., lacerations, abrasions, punctures). These wounds are more prone to infection and require proper cleaning and protection.

Closed Wounds: Skin remains intact but underlying tissue is damaged (e.g., contusions, hematomas). Swelling, pain, and discoloration are common, and complications may include compartment syndrome or deep tissue injury.

3. Types of Open Wounds

Abrasion: Superficial scraping of the skin surface, often caused by friction.

Laceration: Irregular tear in the skin caused by blunt trauma or sharp objects; may have jagged edges.

Incision: A clean, linear wound, commonly surgical in origin. Healing is generally more predictable than in lacerations.

Puncture: A narrow, deep wound caused by a sharp object (e.g., needle, nail). Carries a high risk of infection, particularly if not adequately irrigated.

Avulsion: A forceful detachment of skin and underlying tissue, often producing irregular wound edges and significant tissue loss.

4. Types of Chronic Wounds

Pressure Injuries (formerly Pressure Ulcers): Caused by prolonged pressure, shear, or friction, usually over bony prominences (sacrum, heels). Classified by Stages 1–4, plus unstageable and deep tissue pressure injury (DTPI).

Diabetic Ulcers: Often found on feet; caused by neuropathy, ischemia, and poor circulation. They heal poorly, have a high risk of infection, and may lead to amputation if untreated.

Venous Stasis Ulcers: Occur in the lower legs due to venous insufficiency. Typically shallow with irregular edges, exudate, and hemosiderin staining of surrounding skin. They are often associated with leg swelling and improve with compression therapy.

Arterial Ulcers: Result from poor blood flow due to arterial disease. Painful, often on toes, feet, or ankles; have a "punched-out" appearance with minimal drainage. The surrounding skin is typically cool, pale, and hairless due to poor circulation.

5. Surgical Wounds

- Created intentionally during operative procedures.
- Can be classified as clean, clean-contaminated, contaminated, or infected depending on surgical environment and risk factors.
- Require close monitoring for signs of infection, dehiscence (wound reopening), or delayed healing.

Key Point

Wounds are diverse in etiology, presentation, and healing trajectory. Accurate classification by the clinician is the foundation of effective wound management. This ensures the appropriate selection of dressings, infection control measures, and interventions targeting underlying comorbidities that may impair healing.

CHAPTER 5

Pressure Injury vs. Pressure Ulcer

The term "pressure ulcer" was officially changed to "pressure injury" in 2016 by the National Pressure Ulcer Advisory Panel (NPUAP, now the National Pressure Injury Advisory Panel – NPIAP).

Why the Change Was Made:

1. Accuracy of Description

The word "ulcer" implies an open sore, but in reality, pressure damage can occur under intact skin (for example, Deep Tissue Pressure Injury or Stage 1).

By saying "ulcer," clinicians often overlooked early tissue damage when the skin was not broken.

This sometimes led to delayed intervention and progression of preventable wounds.

2. Inclusive of All Stages

"Pressure injury" covers both situations:

- Skin is intact but damaged (non-blanchable erythema, DTPI).
- Skin is open and ulcerated (Stage 2–4, unstageable).

This inclusivity makes staging more precise and emphasizes that not all pressure-related damage looks the same.

3. Improves Clinical Communication

Using "injury" emphasizes that this is a continuum of tissue damage caused by pressure and shear, not just a surface-level wound.

It also aligns better with how we describe other medical damage (e.g., traumatic injury, brain injury, spinal cord injury).

The broader terminology helps healthcare teams communicate more clearly across disciplines, leading to more consistent treatment plans.

In Summary:

The term was changed to "pressure injury" to make it clearer, more accurate, and inclusive of all stages of pressure-related damage—not just open sores.

The term pressure injury is now preferred over pressure ulcer because it encompasses a wider range of skin damage, according to the American Academy of Family Physicians.

The change in terminology also aligns with international standards and ensures consistency in patient records, education, and clinical guidelines.

Pressure Ulcer Definition

It refers to open ulcerated wounds caused by pressure over a bony prominence. It describes the end result of severe skin breakdown, usually Stage 2 and above.

Pressure Injury

The term is broader, it includes any localized damage to the skin or underlying tissue due to pressure, whether it is an open wound or not.

It includes:

- Intact skin with non-blanchable erythema: Redness that does not turn white when pressed
- Blisters or other skin damage; Even if not yet damaged
- Deep tissue injuries: Injuries that go beyond the skin and may involve muscle, bone, or other tissues.
- Unstageable wounds: Where necrotic tissue or eschar hides the true depth of injury.

Key Takeaway:

Pressure Ulcer = open wound only.

Pressure Injury = all types of damage, from redness to deep necrosis.

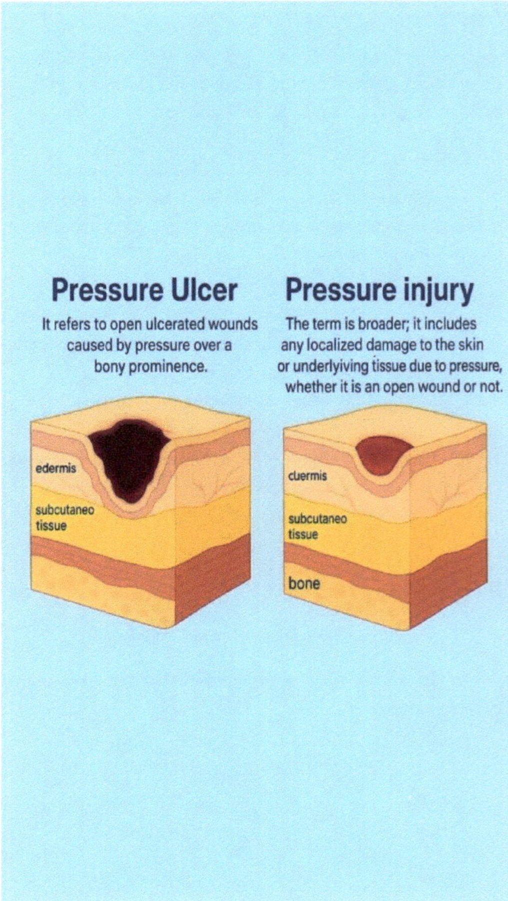
Pressure Ulcer
It refers to open ulcerated wounds caused by pressure over a bony prominence.
edermis
subcutaneo tissue
Pressure injury
The term is broader; it includes any localized damage to the skin or underlyiving tissue due to pressure, whether it is an open wound or not.
cuermis
subcutaneo tissue
bone

CHAPTER 6

Taking an In-Depth Look at Pressure Ulcers

Definition

Pressure ulcers, also known as pressure sores or bed sores, are localized injuries to the skin and underlying tissues that occur due to prolonged pressure, shear, or friction. They are different from other types of wounds in that they are strongly associated with immobility, poor circulation, and prolonged confinement to a bed or chair. Unlike traumatic or surgical wounds, pressure ulcers are preventable but can become chronic and severe if not managed properly.

Cause: Pressure ulcers develop from sustained, unrelieved pressure on a specific area of the body, especially over bony prominences such as the heels, sacrum, hips, or elbows. This pressure reduces blood flow to the tissue, leading to ischemia and cell death.

Tissue Damage: Pressure ulcers often involve progressive skin and underlying tissue destruction, ranging from superficial epidermal damage to full-thickness loss exposing muscle or bone. Visible adipose tissue, granulation tissue, or slough may be present in advanced stages.

Complications: Untreated pressure ulcers can lead to chronic pain, delayed healing, sepsis (blood poisoning), osteomyelitis (bone infection), cellulitis, or even life-threatening systemic infections.

The Stages of Pressure Ulcers

The stages of pressure ulcers are classified into four categories based on severity:

Stage 1: The skin appears red and does not blanch (turn white) when pressed. The area may feel warm, firm, or swollen, but there are no open wounds.

Stage 1: Pressure Ulcer

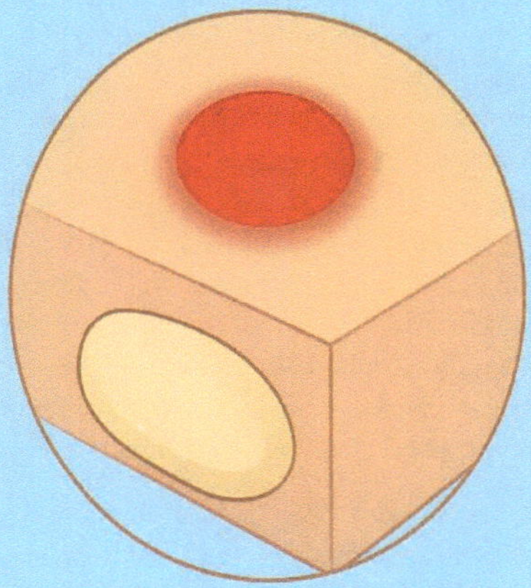

- Skin appears red and does not blanch (turn white) when pressed.
- Area may feel warm, firm, or swollen.
- No open wounds present

Treatment for Stage 1 Pressure Ulcer

To treat Stage 1 pressure ulcers, consider the following steps:

Identify the Cause: Determine the underlying cause of the pressure injury and address it to prevent worsening.

- **Relieve Pressure:** Regularly change positions to relieve pressure on the affected area (e.g., every 1 hour if the patient is emaciated, every 2 hours if the patient is of average weight and size).
- **Maintain Skin Hygiene**: Keep the skin clean, dry, and use moisturizers to prevent dryness.
- **Nutritional Support:** Evaluate and improve the nutritional status of the patient, as proper nutrition aids in healing (e.g., protein and vitamin intake).
- **Monitor Healing:** Stage 1 pressure ulcers can often heal within two to three days if pressure is removed. If not healed after three days, consult a physician.

Stage 2: This stage is characterized by partial-thickness skin loss, resulting in a shallow, open wound that may appear as a blister or erosion.

Stage 2 Pressure Ulcer

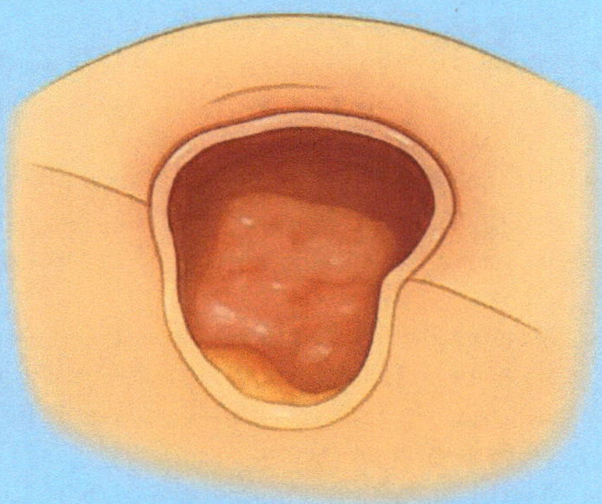

- Partial thickness skin loss
- Shallow open wound
- May look like a blister or crater

Treatment for Stage 2 Pressure Ulcer

The treatment of stage 2 pressure ulcers includes the following steps, which are essential for effective management and healing of stage 2 pressure ulcers.

- **Clean The Wound:** Gently cleanse the ulcer with saline or a mild soap solution to remove debris and bacteria.
- **Apply Dressing:** Use a hydrocolloid or foam dressing to protect the ulcer and maintain a moist environment, which promotes healing.
- **Relieve Pressure:** Implement pressure-relieving strategies, such as repositioning the patient frequently and using specialized mattresses or cushions.
- **Monitor For Infection:** Keep an eye on the ulcer for signs of infection, such as increased redness, swelling, or discharge, and consult a healthcare professional if these occur.
- **Nutritional Support:** Ensure adequate nutrition and hydration to support the healing process.

Stage 3: This stage involves full-thickness loss of skin, where the ulcer extends into the subcutaneous tissue. It may appear as a deep crater and can include necrotic (dead) tissue.

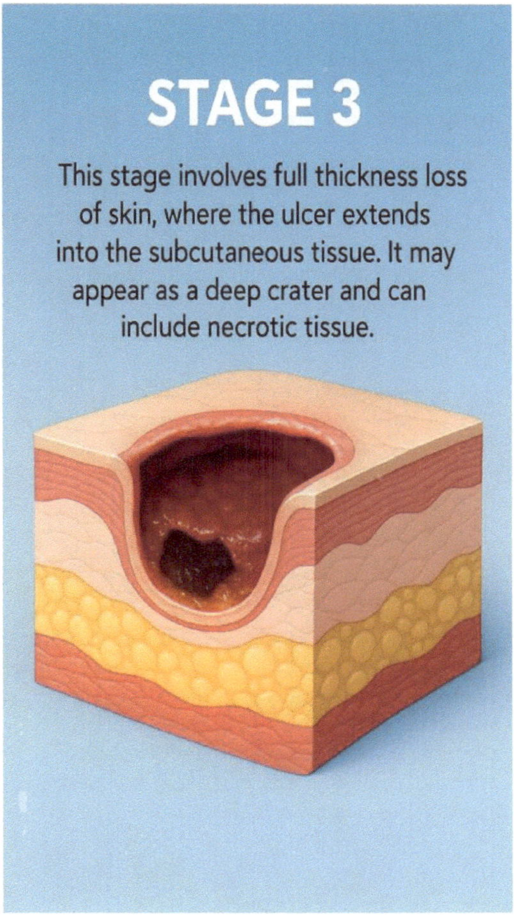
STAGE 3
This stage involves full thickness loss of skin, where the ulcer extends into the subcutaneous tissue. It may appear as a deep crater and can include necrotic tissue.

Treatment for Stage 3 Pressure Ulcer

The treatments aim to facilitate healing and prevent complications associated with stage 3 pressure ulcers. To treat a stage 3 pressure ulcer, consider the following approaches:

- **Address The Ulcer:** Includes antibiotic therapy and removal of dead tissue to promote healing and prevent infection.
- **Wound Debridement:** Properly debride the wound to remove necrotic tissue.
- **Dressings:** Use appropriate dressings such as hydrogel or calcium alginate dressings to maintain moisture and protect the wound.
- **Wound Management:** Manage exudates and keep the wound moist for optimal healing.
- **Ultrasound Therapy:** Consider therapies like non-contact low-frequency ultrasound to promote healing.
- **Consultancy:** Consult a wound specialist for personalized treatment options.

Stage 4: This is the most severe stage, where the ulcer extends through the skin and subcutaneous tissue, exposing muscle, bone, or supporting structures. These treatments aim to promote healing and prevent further complications. Always consult a healthcare professional for personalized care. Slough or eschar may be present, and the risk of serious infection is extremely high.

Stage 4: Pressure Ulcer

Stage 4 is the most severe stage, where the ulcer extends through the skin and subcutaneous tissue, exposing muscle, bone, or supporting structures. These treatments aim to promote healing and prevent further complications. Always consult a healthcare professional for personalized care. This stage carries a high risk of infection.

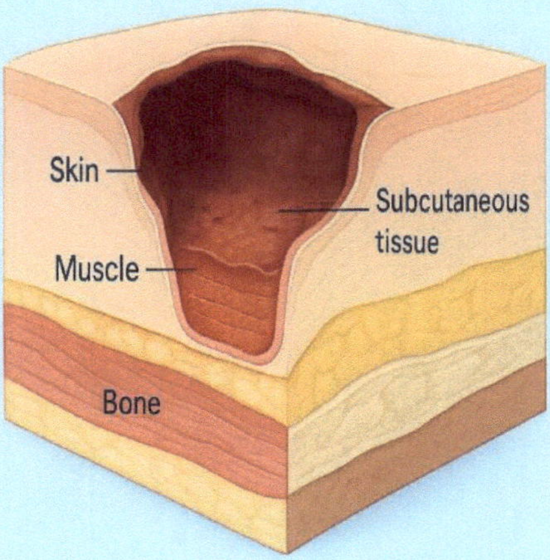

Treatment for Stage 4 Pressure Ulcer

To treat a stage 4 pressure ulcer, consider the following approaches:

- **Immediate Hospitalization:** Patients often require urgent medical attention and may need surgery.
- **Surgical Debridement:** This involves removing damaged, infected, or dead tissue from the ulcer.
- **Antibiotics:** To treat any infections that may be present.
- **Skin Grafts:** Covering the affected area with healthy skin may be necessary.
- **Home and Long-Term Care:** Keeping the area clean, changing positions frequently, and using special support/cushions to relieve pressure are also important.

CHAPTER 7
Taking an In-Depth Look at Arterial Ulcers

Definition

Arterial ulcers or Ischemic ulcers are severe wounds caused by poor blood circulation due to blocked arteries. They primarily develop on the lower extremities, particularly on the feet and toes, where the blood supply is already most vulnerable. Due to their ischemic origin, these ulcers are slow to heal and highly susceptible to infection, often necessitating aggressive medical intervention. These ulcers have a punched-out look with well-defined margins and can lead to serious complications if left untreated.

Taking an In-Depth Look at Arterial ulcers

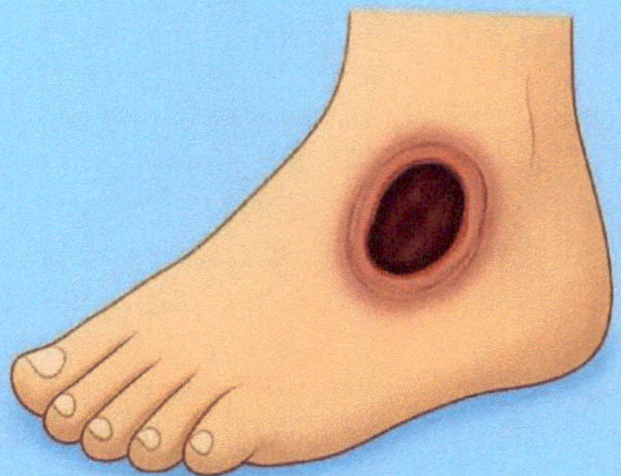

Arterial ulcers or ischemic ulcers are severe wounds caused by poor blood circulation due to blocked arteries.

These ulcers primarily develop on the lower extremities, especially on feet and toes have a punched-out look with well-defined margins, can lead to serious complications if left untreated.

Symptoms

The wounds themselves are characteristically deep, often extending down to the underlying tendons, and will frequently display no signs of new tissue growth. The base of the wound typically does not bleed, and is yellow, brown, grey or black in color. Often, the limb will feel cool or cold to the touch, and the extremity will have little to no distinguishable pulse. The skin and the nails on the extremity will also appear atrophic, with hair loss on the affected extremity, while also taking on a shiny, thin, dry, and taut appearance. In addition, the base color of the extremity may turn red when dangled and pale when elevated.

An additional sign of an arterial ulcer is delayed capillary return in the affected extremity. These ulcers are generally very painful, especially while exercising, at rest, or during the night. A common source of temporary relief from this pain is dangling the affected legs over the edge of the bed, allowing gravity to aid blood flow to the ulcerous region. Arterial ulcers are distinguishable from venous ulcers in that venous ulcers present with redness and edema (swelling) at the site of the ulcer and may be painless.

Etiology

The most common causes of arterial ulcers are:

- Restrictions to blood vessels due to peripheral vascular disease
- Chronic vascular insufficiency
- Vasculitis (inflammatory damage of blood vessels)
- Diabetes mellitus

- Renal failure
- High blood pressure
- Arteriosclerosis (hardening of the arteries)
- Atherosclerosis (thickening of the arteries, due to the buildup of fatty materials)
- Trauma
- Limited joint mobility
- Tobacco use
- Advancing age and general vascular degeneration

Risk Factors

A few risk factors may contribute to the development of an arterial ulcer, including the following comorbidities and conditions:

- Diabetes mellitus
- Foot deformity and callus formation resulting in focal areas of high pressure
- Poor footwear that inadequately protects against high pressure and shear
- Obesity
- Absence of protective sensation due to peripheral neuropathy
- Limited joint mobility
- Advancing age and general vascular degeneration

Complications

If untreated, arterial ulcers can lead to serious complications, including infection, tissue necrosis, and in extreme cases, amputation and significant loss of mobility of the affected limb.

Diagnostic Studies

- Transcutaneous oxygen measurement
- Toe-Brachial Index
- Absolute Toe Systolic Pressure
- Arteriography
- Buerger's test
- Arterial Doppler studies

Treatment of Arterial Ulcers

The following precautions can help minimize the risk of developing arterial ulcers in at-risk patients and minimize complications in patients already exhibiting symptoms:

- Examine feet (especially between the toes) and legs daily for any unusual changes in color or the development of sores.
- Quit smoking. Smoking can harden or clog the arteries, leading to improper perfusion to the extremities.
- Manage blood pressure, cholesterol, triglyceride, and glucose levels.
- Ensure that footwear is properly fitted to avoid points of rubbing or pressure. Avoid wearing constrictive socks.
- Avoid crossing legs while sitting.
- Avoid sitting or standing for extended periods.
- Avoid cold temperatures
- Protect legs and feet from injury and infection.

- Encourage graded physical activity to promote venous return

The primary goal of the treatment of arterial ulcers is to increase circulation to the area, either surgically or medically.

Surgical options range from revascularization to restore normal blood flow to amputation and rehabilitation in patients who cannot be revascularized.

As for non-surgical measures, modifying contributing factors can slow or stop the progression of local ischemia. Additionally, there are boots and pumps available to augment perfusion to the affected limb. The arterial ulcers themselves differ from other severe wounds in that the wound environment should be as dry as possible to decrease the risk of infection.

The use of Cadexomer iodine around the wound margins is an option due to its absorptive properties. This polymer draws exudate and particulate matter from the wound, then, when moist, it releases iodine, serving the dual purpose of cleansing the wound and fighting bacteria at the wound site. Topical antibiotic ointments, such as bacitracin and triple antibiotic, should be used sparingly as they can be toxic to cells.

CHAPTER 8

Taking an In-Depth Look at Venous Stasis Ulcer

Definition

Venous Stasis Ulcers are stubborn wounds caused by chronic venous insufficiency, a condition where the valves in the leg veins are weakened or damaged, making it hard for the legs to manage blood flow effectively. They occur in the lower legs, usually between the knee and ankle, and can cause pain and swelling. If left untreated, they can persist for months or even years, significantly affecting a patient's quality of life. These ulcers form because of blood flow problems in the leg veins, which leads to increased pressure, fluid buildup, and damage to surrounding skin tissues.

Taking an In-Depth look at Venous Stasis Ulcer

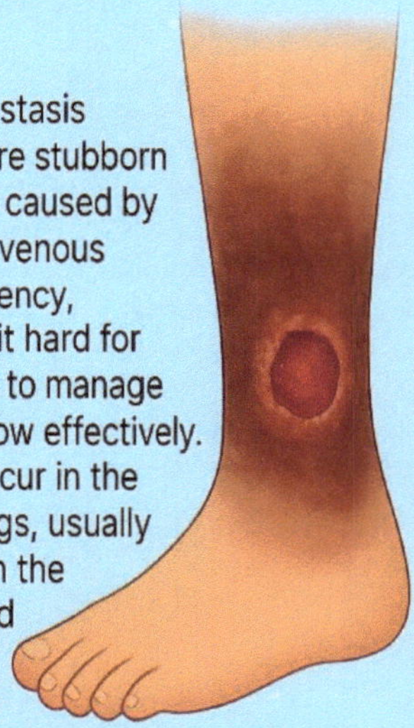

Venous stasis ulcers are stubborn wounds caused by chronic venous insufficiency, making it hard for the legs to manage blood flow effectively. They occur in the lower legs, usually between the knee and ankle, and can cause pain and swelling. These ulcers form because of blood flow problems in the leg vein.

Symptoms

The following symptoms are often present before venous ulcers form.

- Leg cramps and swelling
- Skin becomes thick or hard and changes to dark colors, usually red, purple or brown.
- Tingling and itching of the affected area (this is called stasis dermatitis).
- Varicose veins are a common sign of developing vein problems.
- A feeling of heaviness or tiredness in the legs that improves with elevation.

Stasis ulcers tend to have these symptoms:

- Ulcers tend to form near the ankle.
- The ulcers are shallower and may be red with a yellow layer covering them.
- Ulcers have irregular shapes and the edges are uneven.
- The area around the ulcer can be shiny, and atrophic in appearance. The area is often warmer than the skin further away.
- The ulcers are painful and may bleed or ooze. If they're infected, they may have a foul smell and purulent drainage.

Treatment of Venous Stasis Ulcer

Vascular ulcers may be treated in a variety of ways, depending on how severe they are and what caused them.

Treatment is usually long-term and requires a combination of medical, surgical, and lifestyle-based approaches.

Medications that may be used include:

- **Antibiotics:** Treat an infection. In some cases (such as after surgery), they may be given to prevent an infection from setting in.
- **Topical Gels and Ointments:** Help remove dead or infected tissue, improve circulation to the affected area, prevent infection and help speed up wound healing.
- **Medications to Treat the Underlying Problem:** Controlling your blood pressure and cholesterol, quitting tobacco, and managing your blood sugar can all help wounds heal.
- **Pain Medications or Numbing Agents:** Vascular ulcers and some of the treatments used for them can be painful. It is common for pain or numbing medications to be used during your treatment.
- **Bandages or Types of Wearable Items:** Commonly used to treat vascular ulcers. Use under medical supervision to avoid exacerbating venous hypertension. Misusing these can make a vascular ulcer much worse rather than better.
- **Bandaging:** Covering the ulcer with a protective bandage can help keep it from being infected. Certain

types of bandages may also be medicated, helping speed up wound healing.

- **Compression Garments:** Includes socks, stockings and various other items. By applying pressure to the entire leg, swelling can be limited or stopped. This is commonly used with venous ulcers and helps keep blood from pooling in the legs and feet.
- **Specialized Shoes, Socks or Orthotic Devices**: Many vascular ulcers, especially diabetic ulcers, are caused by simple wear and pressure. Normally, feeling pain from this would cause you to change how you walk, easing the damage to the affected area. However, this doesn't happen with diabetic ulcers because these are often caused by a partial or total loss of feeling in the feet.
- **Moist Wound Dressings:** Maintaining a moist wound environment can help accelerate the healing process while preventing scab formation.

Advanced methods for treating vascular ulcers, especially ones that are larger or are taking longer to heal, may also be used.

- **Revascularization:** Vascular ulcers may happen because of blockages in crucial blood vessels. Revascularization treatments attempt to remove the blockage, helping existing wounds heal and preventing new ones from happening.
- **Surgery:** For wounds that are infected or that are larger and harder to heal, surgery may be used. A surgeon can debride a vascular ulcer to remove dead or infected areas of the wound and perform surgery

to make it easier for the wound to heal. This can include skin grafts and other types of reparative techniques. (In the case of advanced gangrene or very severe vascular ulcers, it is sometimes necessary to amputate part of a foot or leg. This option is meant to save lives and avoid even worse complications. Unfortunately, for people with diabetes, the risk of developing gangrene in the feet is 30 times higher than it is for the average population.)

- **Prescribed Walking:** Physical activity, especially when done with medical guidance, can help improve circulation and help with preventing new vascular ulcers from forming.
- **Hyperbaric Oxygen Therapy:** The normal oxygen level around you is 21%. Hyperbaric oxygen therapy places you in a chamber that has 100% oxygen concentration and higher atmospheric pressure. These conditions can speed up wound healing, especially for vascular ulcers.
- **Debridement:** Dead and infected tissue in and around a vascular ulcer can slow recovery and lead to gangrene and other dangerous complications. Debriding the area removes dead or infected tissue so that only healthy tissue remains.
- **Nutritional Therapy:** A diet rich in protein, vitamins (especially vitamin C and zinc), and hydration is essential to promote faster healing.

CHAPTER 9
Surgical Wounds

What is a Surgical Wound?

A surgical wound is an intentional cut or incision made in the skin and underlying tissues by a surgeon during an operative procedure. Unlike traumatic wounds, which are accidental, surgical wounds are planned and controlled, created under sterile conditions to provide access to internal structures or to remove diseased tissue.

Surgical wounds vary in size and depth depending on the type of surgery (minor skin excision vs. major abdominal surgery). They may be closed primarily with sutures, staples, or adhesive strips, or left partially open to heal by secondary intention in cases of infection risk. The healing process usually occurs in phases: hemostasis, inflammation, proliferation, and remodeling — and each phase can be affected by patient health, wound care, and external factors.

SURGICAL WOUND

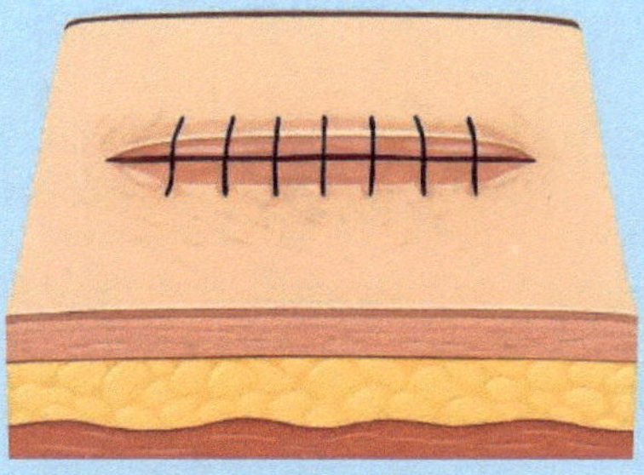

A surgical wound is an intentional cut or incision made in the skin and underlying tissues by a surgeon during an operative procedure. Unlike traumatic wounds, which are accidental, surgical wounds are planned and controlled, created under sterile conditions to provide access to internal structures or to remove diseased tissue.

Surgical wounds vary in size and depth depending on the type of surgery (minor skin excision vs, major abdominal surgery). They may be closed primarily with sutures, staples, or adhesive strips, or left partially open to heal by secondary intention in cases of infection ris. The healing process usually occurs in phases: hemostasis, inflammation, proliferation, and remodeling – and each phase can be affected by patient health,

Causes of Surgical Wounds

1. Planned Surgical Procedures:

- Diagnostic (e.g., biopsy)
- Curative (e.g., tumor removal, appendectomy)
- Reconstructive (e.g., plastic surgery, skin grafts)
- Transplant procedures

2. Accidental or Emergent Surgery:

- Trauma cases requiring operative repair

3. Minimally Invasive Approaches:

- Laparoscopy
- Arthroscopy

Treatment of Surgical Wounds

Treatment goals are to promote healing, prevent infection, and minimize scarring. The approach depends on the wound type, patient's overall condition, and whether complications are present.

1. Wound Closure

- Primary closure (sutures, staples, surgical glue/strips) – most common.
- Secondary intention – wound left open to heal naturally, often for contaminated or infected wounds.
- Tertiary intention (delayed closure) – initially left open, then closed once the risk of infection subsides.

2. Dressing and Protection

- Sterile dressings are applied to absorb exudate, protect against infection, and maintain a moist healing environment.
- Dressing choice depends on wound type (e.g., gauze, hydrocolloid, foam).
- Negative pressure wound therapy (wound VAC) may also be used for large, complex surgical wounds to speed healing and reduce infection risk.

3. Infection Prevention

- Strict aseptic technique during closure.
- Prophylactic antibiotics in high-risk surgeries (e.g., abdominal, orthopedic).
- Hand hygiene and patient education.

4. Patient Care

- Monitoring for signs of infection (redness, swelling, purulent drainage).
- Pain management.
- Nutrition support (adequate protein, vitamins C & A, zinc).
- Blood sugar control in diabetic patients.
- Smoking discontinuation
- Activity restrictions (avoid heavy lifting to protect the wound)

Complications of Surgical Wounds

Despite sterile technique, surgical wounds may develop complications.

1. Dehiscence

Definition: Partial or complete reopening of a surgical wound due to failed healing of the skin and underlying tissues.

Causes:

- Increased abdominal pressure (coughing, straining, obesity)
- Infection at the wound site
- Poor suturing technique
- Malnutrition or compromised immunity
- Steroid use or chronic diseases (e.g., diabetes)
- Excessive physical activity too soon after surgery

Management:

- **Minor Separation:** Managed with dressings and close observation.
- **Major Dehiscence:** Medical emergency requiring immediate surgical intervention (especially with evisceration – organs protruding).
- **Supportive Measures:** Include abdominal binders or reinforcement of sutures in high-risk patients.

2. Infection

- Redness, warmth, swelling, pain, pus drainage, and fever.
- May delay healing or progress to abscess formation or sepsis.

3. Hematoma/Seroma

- Accumulation of blood or serous fluid under the incision site.
- May require drainage.

4. Hypertrophic Scarring or Keloid Formation

- Overproduction of collagen during healing.
- Cosmetic but sometimes functionally restrictive.

5. Adhesions

- Internal scarring leading to bands of fibrous tissue that may cause obstruction (common in abdominal surgeries).
- Can lead to chronic pain, bowel obstruction, or infertility (in gynecological surgeries).

Summary

Surgical wounds are intentional incisions created during operations under sterile conditions. Their healing depends on proper closure, infection prevention, patient health, and post-operative care. While most heal without incident, complications such as infection, hematoma, and dehiscence (the reopening of the wound) may occur. Early detection, prompt management, and patient education are essential to ensure optimal recovery.

CHAPTER 10
Tunneling, Undermining and Rolled Wound Edges

What Causes Tunneling, Undermining, and Rolled Wound Edges

1. Tunneling

Definition: A channel or tract that extends from any part of the wound through subcutaneous tissue or muscle, creating a tunnel-like extension. These hidden pathways often connect different areas of tissue damage, making the wound larger internally than it appears on the surface. Tunnels may be short or extend several centimeters, and they increase the risk of abscess formation, chronic infection, and delayed healing.

Common Causes:

- **Prolonged Pressure:** Common in pressure injuries where deep tissue damage progresses.
- **Infection:** Bacterial spread causes destruction of deeper tissues.
- **Shear and Friction:** Damage between tissue layers encourages tunnel formation.
- **Inadequate Wound Packing:** When wounds are not packed properly, dead spaces allow tissue separation and tunnel formation.

- **Foreign Bodies or Retained Sutures:** Can lead to chronic inflammation and tract formation.
- **Delayed or Improper Wound Care:** Failure to address drainage and pressure points may worsen tunneling.

1. Tunneling

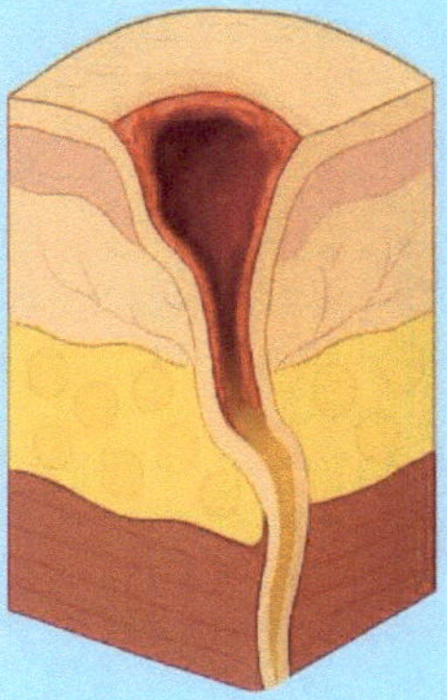

Definition:

A channel or tract that extends from any part of the wound through subcutaneous tissue or muncle, creating a tunnel-like extension.

Common Causes:

- Prolonged Pressure: Common in pressure injuries where deep tissue damage progresses.
- Infection: Bacterial spread causes destruction of deeper tissues.
- Shear and Friction: Damage between tissue layers encourages tunnel formation
- Inadequate Wound Packing: When wounds are not packed properly, dead spaces allow tissue separation
- Foreign Bodies or Retained Sutures: Can lead to chroric inflammation and tract formation

2. Undermining

Definition: Tissue destruction extends under the intact skin around the wound perimeter, creating a shelf or pocket. This makes the wound appear small at the surface but much larger underneath, as the skin edge overhangs the deeper cavity. Undermining weakens wound stability, increases infection risk, and can complicate closure because healthy tissue cannot easily bridge the gap.

Common Causes:

- **Pressure and Shear Forces:** Especially in pressure ulcers, force disrupts connections between tissue layers.
- **Chronic Inflammation:** Persistent inflammation from infection or poor wound management erodes subcutaneous tissue.
- **Ischemia (Poor Perfusion):** Leads to tissue death beneath the skin surface.
- **Infection:** Bacteria can destroy deeper tissue layers while the surface may appear less affected.
- **Trauma or Injury:** Causes deeper tissue disruption without fully breaking the surface skin initially.
- **Inadequate Offloading:** Continued pressure on the wound area delays recovery and promotes undermining.

2. Undermining

Definition:

Tissue destruction extending under the intact skin around w wound perimeter, creating a shelf or pocket.

Common Causes:

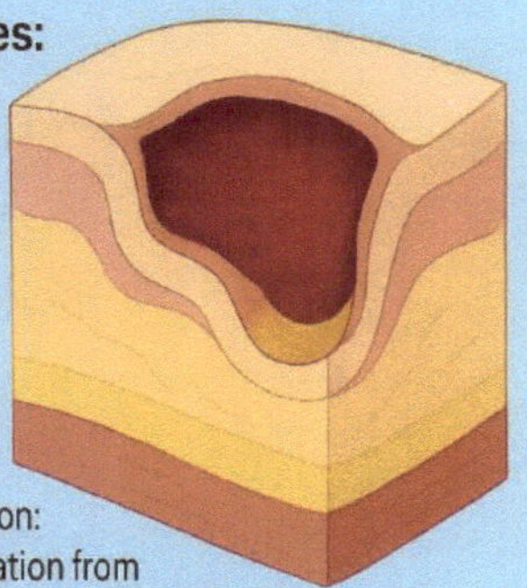

- Pressure and Shear Forces: Especially in pressure uicers force disrupts connections between tissue layers.
- Chronic Inflammation: Persistent inflammation from infection or poor wound management erodes subcutaneous tissue.
- Ischemia (Poor Perfusion): Leads to tissue death beneath the skin surface.
- Infection: Bacteria can destroy deeper tissue layers while the surface may appear less affected.
- Trauma or Injury: Causes deeper tissue disruption without fully breaking the surface skin initially

3. Rolled or Folded Wound Edges (Epibole)

Definition: The wound edges become rolled under and thickened, preventing epithelial cells from migrating across the wound to close it. Instead of advancing across the wound bed, the skin curls inward, essentially "sealing off" the edges. This halts the healing process, traps bacteria or debris inside, and often indicates that the wound has stalled in the inflammatory phase. Epibole typically develops in chronic, non-healing wounds.

Common Causes:

- **Chronic Wound State:** Long-standing wounds often develop Epibole due to stalled healing.
- **Lack of Moisture Balance:** Over-drying or excessive moisture can interrupt normal epithelialization.
- **Non-viable Tissue at the Edges:** Presence of slough, necrosis, or biofilm that impedes new tissue growth.
- **Insufficient Debridement:** Dead tissue or poorly prepared wound bed fails to stimulate proper edge migration.
- **Pressure:** Continuous pressure around the wound edge can prevent proper cell migration and cause the skin to fold inward.
- **Improper Dressing Use:** Dressings that are too dry, too moist, or not changed as recommended can contribute to rolled edges.

Rolled or Folded Wound Edges (Epibole)

Definition: The wound edges become roled under and thickened, preventing epithelial cells from migrating across the wound to close it.

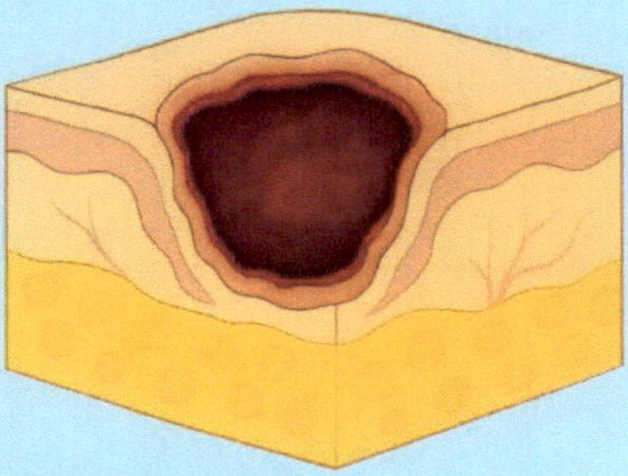

Common Causes:

- Chronic Wound State: Long-standing wounds often develop epibole due to stalled healing
- Lack of Moisture Balance: Over-drying or excessive moisture can interrupt normal epithelialization
- Non-viable Tissue at the Edges: Presence ofslough, necrosis, or biofilm that impedes new tissue growth
- Insufficient Debridement: Dead tissue or poorly prepared wound bed fails to stimulate proper edge migration

Summary of Contributing Factors

Condition	Primary Causes
Tunneling	Pressure, infection, shear, improper packing
Undermining	Pressure/shear, infection, ischemia, chronic inflammation
Rolled Edges	Chronicity, moisture imbalance, necrotic tissue, inadequate debridement

Clinical Note

These conditions indicate impaired wound healing and require:

- Thorough assessment and documentation.
- Debridement if necrotic tissue is present.
- Moisture management to balance exudate.
- Pressure redistribution to prevent further tissue damage.
- Infection control if biofilm or infection is present.
- Nutritional optimization, including protein, vitamins (A, C, zinc), and hydration to support tissue repair.

How To Treat Tunneling, Undermining, And Rolled Wound Edge

1. Tunneling Wounds

Definition: Tunneling occurs when a channel extends from any part of the wound bed into the surrounding tissue, creating a narrow tract.

Treatment Approach:

- **Assessment:** Use a sterile cotton swab to gently measure the depth and direction of tunnels. Document location (using clock method). Regular mapping of tunnels over time is important to monitor progression.
- **Cleansing:** Irrigate the tunnel with normal saline or an appropriate wound cleanser to reduce debris and bacteria. Low-pressure irrigation is recommended to avoid tissue damage.
- **Packing:** Lightly pack with sterile, flexible materials (e.g., alginate rope, gauze, or hydrofiber ribbon) to prevent premature closure at the surface while allowing healing from the base outward.
- **Moisture Balance:** Avoid overpacking (can impair circulation). Dressing should maintain a moist wound environment.
- **Infection Monitoring:** Watch closely for odor, purulent drainage, or systemic infection signs.
- **When to escalate:** If tunnels are >2 cm deep, worsening, or producing copious drainage → surgical consult or advanced therapies (NPWT, debridement).

Tunneling:

Definition:

Tunneling occurs when a channel extends from any part of the wound bed into the surrounding tissue, creating a narrow tract.

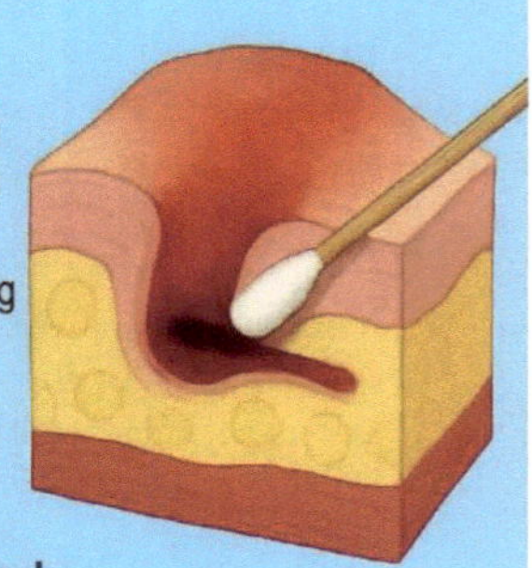

Treatment Approach:

- **Assessment:** Use a sterile cotton swab to gently measure the depth and direction of tunnels. Document location (using clock method).
- **Cleansing:** Irrigate the tunnel with normal saline or an appropriate wound cleanser to reduce debris and bacteria.
- **Packing:** Lightly pack with sterile, flexible materials (e.g., alginate rope, gauze, or hydrofiber ribbon) to prevent premature closure at the surface while allowing healing from the base outward.
- **Moisture Balance:** Avoid overpacking (can impair circulation). Dressing should maintain a moist wound environment.
- **Infection Monitoring:** Watch closely for odor, purulent drainage, or systemic infection signs.

2. Undermining Wounds

Definition: Undermining is tissue destruction under the intact skin around the wound's edges, creating a "lip" or shelf.

Treatment Approach:

- **Assessment:** Probe under the wound edge using the clock method (e.g., undermining from 2 o'clock to 5 o'clock, depth 2 cm).
- **Debridement:** Remove non-viable tissue if present (per scope of practice—sharp, enzymatic, or autolytic).
- **Packing:** Fill the undermined space with packing material to eliminate dead space (calcium alginate, collagen, hydrofiber, or NPWT foam).
- **Pressure Redistribution:** For pressure injuries, offload pressure (specialty mattress, repositioning). Strict turning schedules every 2 hours are essential in bedbound patients.
- **Monitor Edges:** Prevent edge collapse with appropriate dressing support and wound stabilization.
- **When to Escalate:** Rapid progression of undermining, suspected abscess, or osteomyelitis. If bone is exposed or palpable, urgent referral is required.

Definition:

Undermining is tissue destruction under the intact skin around the wound's edges, creating a 'lip" or shelf.

Treatment Approach:

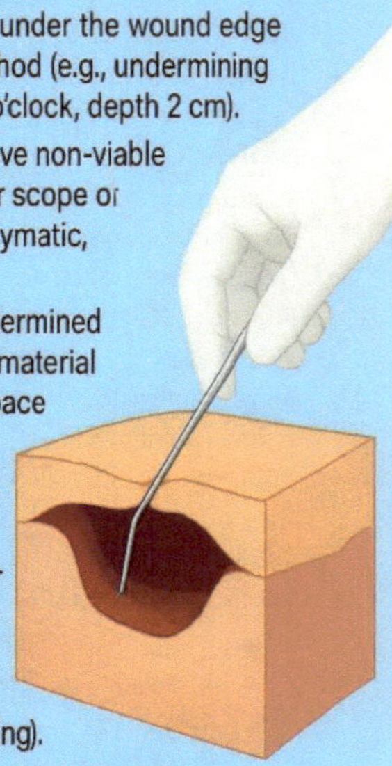

- Assessment: Probe under the wound edge using the clock method (e.g., undermining from 2 o'clock to 5 o'clock, depth 2 cm).
- Debridement: Remove non-viable tissue if present (per scope or practice -sharp, enzymatic, or autolytic).
- Packing: Fill the undermined space with packing material to eliminate dead space (calcium alginate, collagen, hydrofiber, or NPWT foam).
- Pressure Redistribution: For pressure injuries, offload pressure (speciialty mattress, repositioning).
- Monitor Edges: Prevent progression of undermining, suspected abscess, or osteomyelitis.

3. Rolled Wound Edges (Epibole)

Definition: Epibole occurs when wound edges roll under and epithelial cells stop migrating—stalls wound closure.

Treatment Approach:

- **Debridement:** Non-viable, rolled tissue should be debrided (sharp, mechanical, or chemical) to re-expose the wound edge.
- **Edge Stimulation:** Some clinicians use silver nitrate sticks or mechanical debridement to encourage fresh epithelialization.
- **Moisture Balance:** Use dressings that keep the wound moist but not macerated (hydrocolloids, hydrogels, foams).
- **Adjunct Therapy:** Consider NPWT or biological agents (collagen matrix, growth factor dressings) if the wound fails to progress.
- **Nutritional & Systemic Support:** Ensure adequate protein, hydration, and control of comorbidities (e.g., diabetes, vascular disease).
- **When to Escalate:** Chronic wounds with persistent Epibole despite interventions should be referred to a wound care specialist.

Rolled Wound Edges (Epibole)

Definition:

Epibole occurs when wound edges roll under and epithelial cells stop migrating--stalls wound closure.

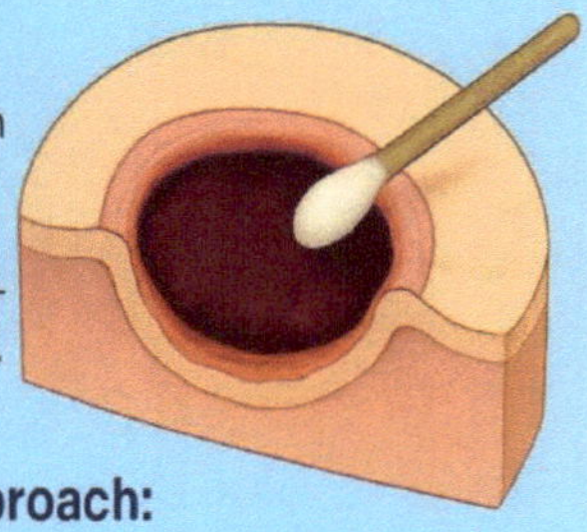

Treatment Approach:

Debridement: Non-viaile, rolled tissue shuuld be debrided (sharp, mechanical, or chemical) to encour age fresh epithelialization.

Moisture Balance: Use dressings that keep wound moist but not macerated (hydrocolloids, hydrogels, toams).

Adjunct Therapy: Consider NPWT or biological agents (collagen matrix, growth factor dressings) if wound fails to progress.

Nutritional& Systemic Support: Ensure adequate protein, hydration, and control of comorbidities (e.g. diabetes, vascular disease).

When to escalate: Chronic wounds with persistent epibole despite interventions should be referred to a wound care specialist.

Quick Reference Summary

Complication	Treatment Focus
Tunneling	Cleanse & lightly pack tunnels, prevent premature closure, monitor infection
Undermining	Fill undermined space, debride devitalized tissue, offload pressure
Rolled Edges	Debride rolled tissue, stimulate edge regrowth, maintain moisture balance

Important: Always base interventions on wound etiology (pressure, diabetic, venous, arterial, surgical, etc.) and patient comorbidities. Advanced or non-healing wounds should be referred to a wound care specialist or WOCN for further management.

CHAPTER 11
Wound Measurement

Wound Measurement Method (Length × Width × Depth + Tunneling/Undermining)

Preparation and Equipment

Supplies: Non-sterile gloves, normal saline, gauze, wound ruler (cm and inches), sterile cotton-tipped applicator(s), flashlight, new dressing, disposal bag.

Analgesia: Give pain meds per order 30–45 min before if needed. Topical lidocaine gel or soaked gauze may also be considered for highly painful wounds.

Asepsis: Remove the old dressing, cleanse first, then measure (odor is only meaningful after cleansing). Always perform hand hygiene before and after, and follow standard precautions to reduce infection risk.

Units & Conversions:

- Use cm as your primary unit.
- Add inches as needed.
- cm → in: divide by 2.54
- in → cm: multiply by 2.54

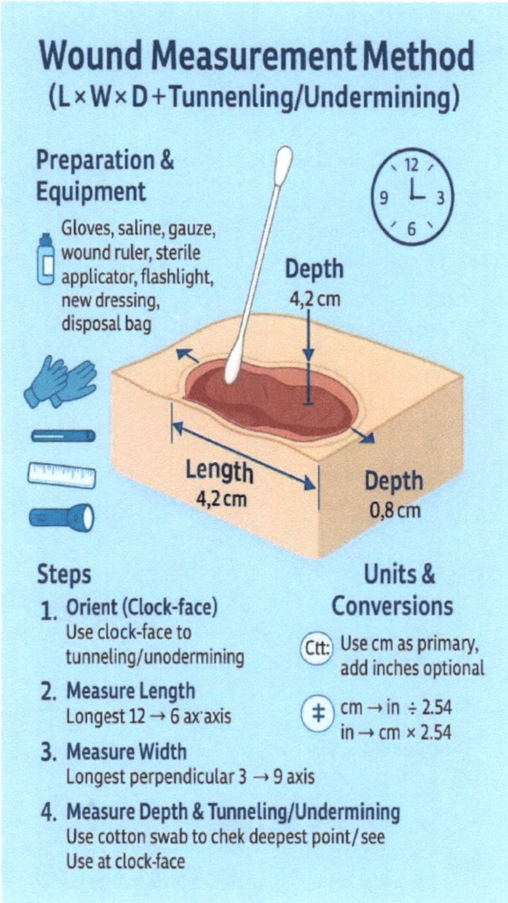
Wound Measurement Method
(L × W × D + Tunnenling/Undermining)
Preparation & Equipment
Gloves, saline, gauze, wound ruler, sterile applicator, flashlight, new dressing, disposal bag
12
9
3
6
Depth
4,2 cm
Length
4,2 cm
Depth
0,8 cm
Steps
1. Orient (Clock-face)
Use clock-face to tunneling/unodermining
2. Measure Length
Longest 12 → 6 ax axis
3. Measure Width
Longest perpendicular 3 → 9 axis
4. Measure Depth & Tunneling/Undermining
Use cotton swab to chek deepest point/ see
Use at clock-face
Units & Conversions
Ctt:
Use cm as primary, add inches optional
‡
cm → in ÷ 2.54
in → cm × 2.54

1. Orient yourself (the "clock-face" method)

Imagine a clock over the wound:

- 12 o'clock = toward the patient's head
- 6 o'clock = toward the feet.
- Patient's right side is 3 o'clock.

This keeps measurements consistent across staff and visits. This method is critical for wounds with tunneling/undermining, ensuring accurate documentation of direction and reducing variability.

2. Measure Length (L)

Definition: The longest distance from head-to-toe (12→6 o'clock) over intact skin.

- Place the disposable ruler gently across the longest head-to-toe axis.
- Record to the nearest 0.1 cm (and inches if you want both).
- Example: Length = 4.2 cm (1.65 in)

Clinical Note: Avoid stretching the wound or surrounding skin while measuring, as this may exaggerate size.

3. Measure Width (W)

Definition: The longest distance perpendicular to the length (3→9 o'clock).

- Measure across the widest point at a right angle to your length line.
- Record to 0.1 cm (and inches if desired).

- Example: Width = 3.1 cm (1.22 in)

Clinical Note: Always confirm you are measuring perpendicular, not diagonally, to avoid errors.

4. Measure Depth (D)

Definition: Vertical distance from the skin surface to the deepest point of the wound bed.

- Moisten a sterile cotton-tipped applicator with saline. Insert to the deepest point.
- Pinch the applicator at skin level, withdraw, then measure the tip-to-pinch distance on your ruler.
- Example: Depth = 0.8 cm (0.32 in)
- Do not force through eschar or non-yielding slough. If the bed is obscured, chart: "Depth unable to assess due to adherent slough/eschar."

Clinical Note: Multiple depths may exist; record the maximum depth and note the location on the clock face.

5. Assess Tunneling (Sinus tracts)

Definition: A narrow channel extending away from the wound bed.

- Gently probe with a sterile applicator in all directions; never force.
- Record direction by clock and length in cm.
- Example: Tunneling: 2.3 cm at 4 o'clock.

Clinical Note: Tunneling often indicates infection, shear, or abscess formation, always monitor for systemic signs (fever, odor, erythema).

6. Assess Undermining

Definition: A "lip" or shelf of tissue where the wound extends under the intact skin at the edge.

- Insert a moistened sterile applicator under the edge and sweep around the clock.
- Record the clock range and the maximum depth.
- Example: Undermining: from 1–4 o'clock, max 1.2 cm at 3 o'clock.

Clinical Note: Undermining may be extensive even if the wound looks small on the surface, always sweep 360° if possible.

7. Describe the Wound Bed

- Estimate percentages (must total 100%):
    - Granulation (red, pebbled) %
    - Slough (yellow/tan/grey, stringy) %
    - Eschar (brown/black, leathery) %
    - Exposed structures (fat, tendon, bone, fascia, device), if present.
- Example: Bed: 70% granulation, 30% slough; no exposed structures.

Clinical Note: Photographing the wound (with scale and date) greatly improves consistency of % estimates.

8. Document the Edges and Peri-wound skin

- **Edges:** Attached/unattached, Epibole (rolled), callused, macerated, or inflamed.

- **Peri-wound (within ~4 cm of the edge):** Intact vs. maceration, erythema (note width), induration, warmth/coolness, edema, rash, denudement.

Clinical Note: Look for satellite lesions or skin breakdown from adhesives/dressings.

9. Exudate & Odor (after cleansing)

- **Amount:** None, scant, small, moderate, large/copious.
- **Type:** Serous, serosanguineous, sanguineous, purulent (green/yellow, thick).
- **Odor:** None/mild/moderate/strong after cleansing.

Clinical Note: Note changes over time; sudden increase in purulent drainage or odor often signals infection.

10. Pain & Functional Impact

- Pain 0–10 scale at rest and with care; note descriptors (burning, throbbing).
- Function: Offloading needs, gait limits, sleep disruption, and ADL impact.

Clinical Note: Always reassess pain post-procedure and document relief strategies.

11. Area & Volume (optional but useful for tracking)

- **Simple rectangular area (cm^2):** Area $\approx L \times W$
- **Using examples:** $4.2 \times 3.1 = 13.0$ cm^2
- **Elliptical area (cm^2) for curved wounds:** Area $\approx \pi \times (L/2) \times (W/2)$
    - $3.1416 \times 2.1 \times 1.55 \approx 10.2$ cm^2

- **Approximate volume (cm^3):** L × W × D
  - 4.2 × 3.1 × 0.8 ≈ 10.4 cm^3
- **Healing trend:** Track area weekly; consistent decrease indicates progress.

Clinical Note: Use digital wound measurement apps or software when available to increase accuracy.

12. Consistency tips (to reduce inter-rater variability)

- Measure in cm to 0.1 accuracy; add inches for clarity.
- Use the same orientation (12/6 for length, 3/9 for width) every time.
- Ideally, the same clinician measures weekly; if not, ensure the same method.
- Photo (if permitted): include a measurement scale, date/time, and consistent angle/lighting (protect privacy/HIPAA).

Sample Documentation (Complete, Concise)

Location: Left lateral malleolus.

L×W×D: 4.2 cm × 3.1 cm × 0.8 cm (≈ 1.65 in × 1.22 in × 0.32 in).

Area (L×W): 13.0 cm^2; Volume (L×W×D): 10.4 cm^3.

Tunneling: 2.3 cm at 4 o'clock.

Undermining: 1–4 o'clock, max 1.2 cm at 3 o'clock.

Bed: 70% granulation, 30% slough, no exposed structures.

Edges: Partially unattached; no Epibole.

Peri-wound: Mild erythema 1.0 cm wide; no induration, no maceration.

Exudate: Moderate serosanguineous; odor none after cleansing.

Pain: 3/10 at rest, 5/10 with care.

Plan: Continue offloading; consider enzymatic debridement; reassess in 7 days.

Common Pitfalls (And Fixes)

- Measuring before cleansing → overcalls odor/exudate. Always cleanse first.
- Switching axes between visits → trend becomes meaningless. Use 12–6 for length every time.
- Forcing a probe → trauma/bleeding. Stop if resistance/pain.
- Estimating percentages → wide variability. Round to the nearest 5–10% and be consistent.
- Reverse staging pressure injuries → Never reverse-stage; just measure and describe healing.

Conversion Reference

- 2.0 cm = 0.79 in
- 5.0 cm = 1.97 in
- 10.0 cm = 3.94 in

CHAPTER 12

Case Studies and Sample Documentation

Diabetic Foot Ulcer

Case Study

Mr. L, a 62-year-old male with a 15-year history of poorly controlled Type 2 Diabetes Mellitus, presented with a non-healing wound on the plantar surface of his right foot. The wound measured 3.0 cm x 2.5 cm with a depth of 0.7 cm, showing moderate serosanguinous drainage and surrounding callus formation. The patient reported diminished sensation in both feet, consistent with peripheral neuropathy. Poor glycemic control, combined with loss of protective sensation, contributed to repeated trauma and delayed healing. Interventions included debridement of necrotic tissue, offloading with a specialized shoe insert, tight glucose monitoring, and education on daily foot inspection. After six weeks of coordinated wound care and improved diabetes management, the ulcer showed granulation tissue formation and reduced size, although long-term risk for recurrence remained high.

Case Study: Diabetic Foot Ulcer

Mr. L. a 62-year-old male with a 15-year history of poorly controlled Type 2 Diabetes Mellitus, presented with a no-nealing wound on plantar surface of his right foot. Showing moderate serosanguinuous drainage and surrounding callus formation. The patiert reports diminished sensation in both feet, consistent with n peripheral neuropathy, Poor glycemic control combined with loss of protective sensaction led to repeated trauma and delayed healing. long-tarm risk for recurrence remained high.

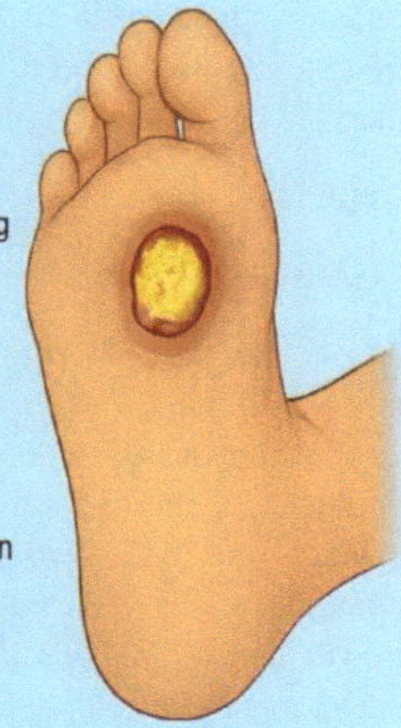

Sample Documentation of Diabetic Foot Ulcer

Diabetic Ulcer

Right plantar foot wound measuring 3.0 cm x 2.5 cm x 0.7 cm. Wound bed 60% pale granulation, 40% yellow siough. Surrounding callus noted. Moderate serosanguinous drainage with no foul odor. Peri-wound skin intact but dry. Patient reports no pain due to neuropathy. Dressing applied: moist-to-dry with protective offloading boot. Patient educated on daily foot inspection and glucose monitoring.

Sample Documentation of Diabetic Foot Ulcer

Right plantar foot wound measuring 3.0 cm x 2.5 cm x 0.7 cm. Wound bed 60% pale granulation, 40% yellow slough. Surrounding callus noted. Moderate serosanguinous drainage with no foul odor. Peri-wound skin is intact but dry. Patient reports no pain due to neuropathy. Dressing applied: moist-to-dry with protective offloading boot. Patient educated on daily foot inspection and glucose monitoring.

Arterial Ulcer

Case Study

Mrs. J, a 71-year-old female with a history of peripheral arterial disease and hypertension, was evaluated for a painful ulcer on her left lateral ankle. The wound measured 2.0 cm x 1.5 cm, with a pale wound bed, minimal exudate, and well-demarcated, punched-out edges. The surrounding skin was cool to the touch with reduced hair growth, and pedal pulses were weak on palpation. The patient reported intermittent claudication and severe pain at night, relieved by dangling her foot off the bed. Arterial insufficiency was confirmed by an ankle-brachial index of 0.6. Management included referral to vascular surgery for revascularization assessment, pain control, and use of non-adherent dressings to protect the wound. Despite appropriate local wound care, healing was delayed due to compromised perfusion, underscoring the importance of addressing the underlying vascular disease.

Case Study: Arterial Ulcer

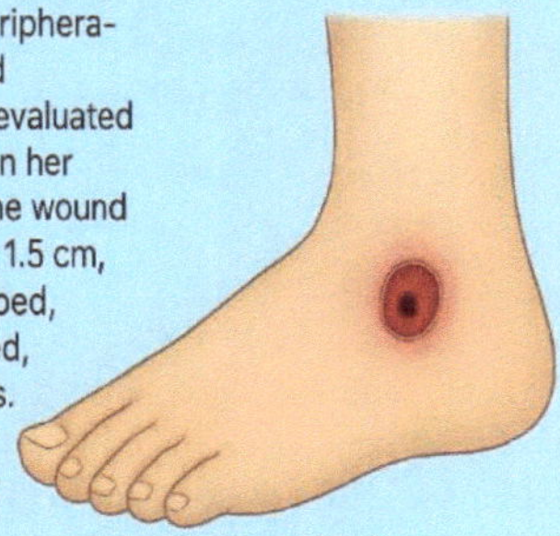

Mrs. J. 71-year old female with a history of periphera-arterial disease and hypertension, was evaluated for a painful ulcer on her left lateral ankle. The wound measured 2.0 cm x 1.5 cm, with a pale wound bed, minimal-dumarcated, punched-out edges. The surrounding skin is cool to toutc with reduced hair growth, and pedal pulses are weak on paalpation. Despite appropriate local wound care, healing was elayed duto compromised perfusion, underscoring the importan-ce of addressing the underlying vascular disease,under-scoring the importance of addressing the underlying vascular disease.

Sample Documentation

Arterial Ulcer

Left lateral ankle wound measuring 2.0 cm x 1 5 cm, depth 0.3 cm Wound bed paie, dry, with minimai granulation tissue. Borders sharply demarcated with "punched-out appcarance. Surrounding skin cool, shiny, hairless. Pedal pulse weak (1+). Patient reports severe pain. 8/10, relieved when leg is dependent.

Sample Documentation of Arterial Ulcer

Left lateral ankle wound measuring 2.0 cm x 1.5 cm, depth 0.3 cm. Wound bed pale, dry, with minimal granulation tissue. Borders are sharply demarcated with a "punched-out" appearance. Surrounding skin is cool, shiny, and hairless. Pedal pulse weak (1+). Patient reports severe pain, 8/10, relieved when the leg is dependent. Minimal serous drainage, no odor. Dressing applied: non-adherent dry sterile dressing. Referral to a vascular surgeon in place.

Venous Stasis Ulcer

Case Study

Mr. T, a 58-year-old male with a history of chronic venous insufficiency and obesity, presented with a shallow ulcer located on the medial aspect of his right lower leg. The ulcer measured 4.5 cm x 3.2 cm, with irregular borders, moderate serous drainage, and a red granulating wound bed. Surrounding skin showed hemosiderin staining, edema, and lipodermatosclerosis. The patient reported aching and heaviness in the leg that worsened after prolonged standing and improved with elevation. Venous Doppler confirmed reflux in the saphenous vein. Treatment included multilayer compression therapy, leg elevation, wound cleansing, and patient education on weight management and mobility exercises. Over eight weeks, the ulcer gradually reduced in size, highlighting the effectiveness of compression in managing venous stasis disease.

Case Study: Venous Stasis Ulcer

Mr. T, a 58-year-old male with a history of chronic venous insufficiency and hypertension, presented with a shallow ulcer located on the medial aspect of his right lower leg. Treatment included mulitlayer compression therapy, leg elevation, wound cleansing and patient education on weight management arind mobility exercises.
Over eight weeks the ulcer. gradually reduced in size, highlighting theffective-ness of compression in managing venous stasis disease.

Before Compression

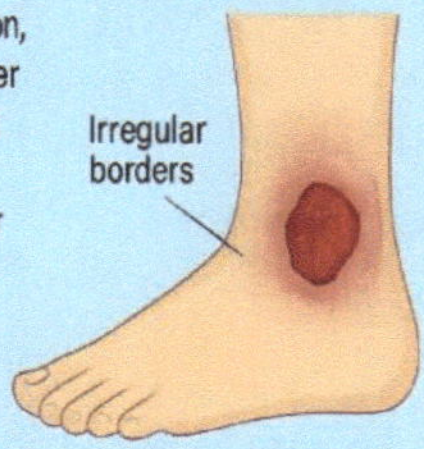

After 8 Weeks Compression

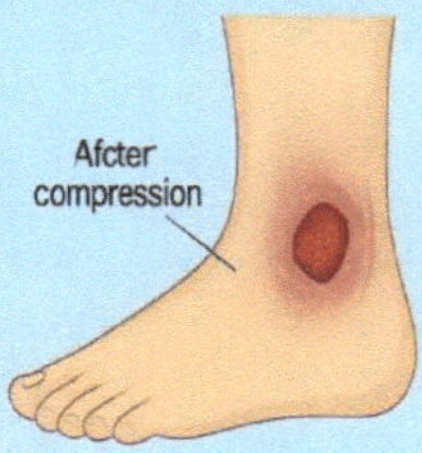

Sample Documentation

Right medial lower leg wound measuring 4.5 cm x 3.2 cm, depth 0.4 cm. Wound bed beffy red with 70% granulation, 30% olough. Moderate serous drania-ge with no foul odor. Irregular wound borders. Surrounding skin hyperpigmented with hemosiderin staning, +2 pitting e-dema, Patient reports mild aching, 4/10, worse after standing.

Sample Documentation of Venous Stasis Ulcer

Right medial lower leg wound measuring 4.5 cm x 3.2 cm, depth 0.4 cm. Wound bed beefy red with 70% granulation, 30% slough. Moderate serous drainage with no foul odor. Irregular wound borders. Surrounding skin hyperpigmented with hemosiderin staining, +2 pitting edema. Patient reports mild aching, 4/10, worse after standing. Compression bandaging applied. Patient instructed to elevate legs when resting.

Surgical Wound

Case Study

Ms. P, a 46-year-old female, underwent an open cholecystectomy and developed a surgical wound along the right upper quadrant measuring 8.0 cm in length. On post-operative day 5, the wound edges were partially separated, with scant serosanguinous drainage noted. The wound bed appeared clean with early granulation tissue, and sutures remained intact along the majority of the incision. The patient denied fever or chills but reported mild tenderness around the site. Risk factors included obesity and mild diabetes, which may have contributed to delayed primary healing. Interventions included reinforcement of sterile dressings, reinforcement of glycemic control, and continued monitoring for infection. Over the next two weeks, with regular wound care and improved nutritional intake, the incision site gradually closed and healed without further complication.

Case Study: Surgical Wound

Ms. P, a 46-year-old female, underwent an open cholecystectomy and developed a surgical wound along the right upper quadrant measuring 8.0 cm in length. On post-operative day 5, the wound edges were partially separated, with scant serosanguinuos drainage noted. The wound bed appeared elean with early granulation tissue, and sutures remained intact along the majority of the incision.
The patient denied fever or chills but reported mild tenderness around the site, Risk factors included obesity and mild diabctes, which may have contributed to delayed primary healing. Interventions included reinforcement of sterile dressings, reinforcement of glycemic control, and continued monitoring for infection. Over the next two weeks, with regular wound care and improved nutritional intaike, the incision site gradually closed and healed without further complication.

Post-op Day 5 | **After 2 Weeks**

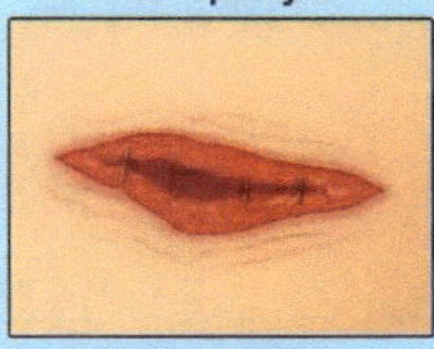

Post op Day 5

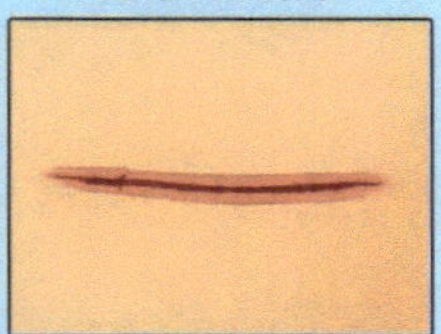

After 2 Weeks

Sample Documentation

Surgical Wound
Right upper quadrant abdominal incision measuring 8.0 cm length, approximated edges with partial dehiscence at mid-point (15 cm)
Wound bed pink with scant granulation tissue. Scant serosanguginioaos drainage, no foul odor. Sutures intact at proximal and distal ends.
Surrounding skin slightly erythematous but non-tender. Patient reports mild

Sample Documentation of Surgical Wound

Right upper quadrant abdominal incision measuring 8.0 cm in length, approximated edges with partial dehiscence at mid-point (1.5 cm). Wound bed pink with scant granulation tissue. Scant serosanguinous drainage, no foul odor. Sutures intact at proximal and distal ends. Surrounding skin is slightly erythematous but non-tender. Patient reports mild pain 3/10. Dressing changed using sterile technique, incision reinforced. Patient advised on signs of infection and the importance of glycemic control.

CHAPTER 13
WOCN-Based Wound Treatment Recommendations

1. Dry Wounds

Goal: Add moisture to facilitate healing.

Recommended Treatments:

- **Hydrogels:** Provide moisture, pain relief, and support autolytic debridement **(e.g., Sheets, Gels).**
- **Hydrocolloids:** Occlusive dressings that maintain a moist environment and protect against external contaminants.
- **Impregnated Gauze with Hydrogel:** Useful for irregularly shaped wounds.
- **Saline-moistened Gauze (short term only):** Not recommended for long-term use due to drying out and risk of adherence to wound bed

2. Moist or Wet Wounds with Moderate to Heavy Exudate

Goal: Absorb excess moisture, manage drainage, prevent maceration.

Recommended Treatments:

- **Calcium Alginate Dressings:** Highly absorbent, ideal for wounds with heavy drainage.

- **Hydrofiber Dressings**: Gel on contact with fluid, conforming closely to the wound bed (e.g., Aquacel).
- **Foam Dressings:** Provide cushioning, thermal insulation, and longer wear time.
- **Composite Dressings:** Combine absorption with bacterial barrier for versatile use.

3. Necrotic Wounds (with Slough or Eschar)

Goal: Debride necrotic tissue.

Recommended Treatments:

- **Enzymatic Debridement:** Selectively targets necrotic tissue without damaging viable tissue (Collagenase).
- **Autolytic Debridement:** Promotes natural enzyme action for gentle debridement (using occlusive dressings like Hydrocolloids, Hydrogels).
- **Sharp/Surgical Debridement:** Fastest method, used when urgent removal of necrosis is required.
- **Mechanical Debridement (used cautiously):** Includes wet-to-dry dressings or wound irrigation; may damage healthy tissue.
- **Biosurgical Debridement:** Effective in resistant cases, maggots secrete enzymes that liquefy necrotic tissue. (Maggot Therapy)

4. Infected Wounds

Goal: Reduce bioburden and control infection.

Recommended Treatments:

- **Antimicrobial Dressings:**

    - Silver-impregnated Dressings: Broad-spectrum antimicrobial effect.
    - Iodine-based Dressings: Absorbs exudate while releasing iodine (e.g., Cadexomer Iodine).
    - PHMB (Polyhexamethylene Biguanide) Dressings: Low-toxicity antimicrobial agent.
    - Honey-impregnated Dressings: Reduce biofilm and promote autolysis (e.g., Manuka Honey).
- **Topical Antibiotics (short-term, targeted):** Only for localized infections.
- **Systemic Antibiotics (as ordered by the physician):** Necessary when there are systemic signs of infection (e.g., fever, spreading cellulitis).

5. Granulating Wounds

Goal: Protect new tissue, maintain a moist wound environment.

Recommended Treatments:

- **Non-adherent Dressings:** Minimize disruption of fragile granulation tissue during dressing changes.
- **Hydrogels:** Keep the wound moist and reduce pain.
- **Foam Dressings:** Absorb excess exudate while maintaining moisture.
- **Hydrocolloids:** Protect the wound and encourage autolytic debridement of residual slough.

6. Epithelializing Wounds

Goal: Protect the fragile new epithelium and prevent trauma.

Recommended Treatments:

- **Transparent Films:** Allow visualization of wound healing while providing a protective barrier.
- **Non-adherent Dressings:** Reduce trauma on removal.
- **Silicone-coated Dressings:** Soft and gentle, suitable for fragile skin.

7. Wounds with Undermining or Tunneling

Goal: Fill dead space, prevent abscess formation.

Recommended Treatments:

- **Packing with Ribbon Gauze or Hydrogel:** Impregnated Gauze: Ensures wound closure from the base upward.
- **Hydrofiber Dressings:** Conform to wound channels, reducing the risk of abscess.
- **Calcium Alginate (if exudative):** Absorbs drainage while filling spaces.

8. Specialty Treatments

- **Negative Pressure Wound Therapy (NPWT):** Applies continuous or intermittent suction to remove exudate, increase blood flow, and stimulate granulation; useful in large, complex, or surgical wounds.
- **For Complex Wounds, Deep Wounds, Or Surgical Dehiscence:**
  Bioengineered Skin Substitutes: Promote closure in chronic non-healing wounds such as diabetic foot

ulcers or venous ulcers.

- **For Non-Healing Chronic Wounds:**
  - Growth Factor Therapy: Used selectively for diabetic foot ulcers, accelerates healing by stimulating cellular activity.

General WOCN Treatment Principles:

- Always maintain a moist wound environment unless contraindicated (e.g., dry stable eschar in ischemic limbs).
- Prevent maceration of surrounding skin with barrier products.
- Reassess wounds regularly for changes in size, depth, exudate, infection, and tissue type.
- Select dressings based on wound type, exudate level, and healing phase.
- Consider patient comfort, pain management, and cost-effectiveness when choosing products.
- Provide education to patients and caregivers regarding wound care, dressing changes, and recognition of early signs of infection.

SAMPLE WOUND DOCUMENTATION TEMPLATE

Patient Information:

Name: ______________________________

MRN: ______________________________

Date: ______________ Time: ______________

Location of Wound: ______________________

Wound Etiology (if known): ☐ Pressure Injury ☐ Diabetic Ulcer ☐ Venous Stasis ☐ Arterial ☐ Surgical ☐ Other: __________

Wound Assessment:

Wound Type/Stage (if pressure injury): __________________

Wound Size:

Length: ______ cm

Width: ______ cm

Depth: ______ cm

Tunneling:

Present? ☐ Yes ☐ No

Location (clock method): __________

Depth: ______ cm

Undermining:

Present? ☐ Yes ☐ No

Location (clock method): __________

Maximum depth: ______ cm

Edges:

☐ Attached ☐ Unattached ☐ Rolled/Epibole ☐ Calloused ☐ Macerated

Wound Bed:

% Granulation Tissue: ______ %

% Slough: ______ %

% Eschar: ______ %

Color/Description: ________________________

EXUDATE/DRAINAGE:

Amount: ☐ None ☐ Scant ☐ Small ☐ Moderate ☐ Large

Type: ☐ Serous ☐ Serosanguinous ☐ Purulent ☐ Other: ___________

Odor: ☐ None ☐ Mild ☐ Moderate ☐ Strong

Surrounding Skin:

☐ Intact ☐ Redness ☐ Induration ☐ Warmth ☐ Maceration ☐ Excoriation

Pain Assessment:

☐ No pain ☐ Mild ☐ Moderate ☐ Severe

Patient reported pain level (0–10): ____

Treatment/Interventions:

Cleansing solution: ____________________

Debridement performed? ☐ Yes ☐ No (type:____________)

Packing Material Used (If Applicable):

____

Primary dressing: ____________________

Secondary dressing: ____________________

Offloading device/pressure redistribution: ☐ Yes ☐ No (type: ____________)

Additional interventions:

____

Evaluation & Plan:

Wound response to treatment:

____

Next due dressing change: ____________________

Referrals needed: ☐ WOCN ☐ Physician ☐ Surgeon ☐ Other: ___________

Education Provided to Patient/Caregiver:

____

Nurse Signature/Title: ________________________

This template ensures completeness, compliance, and clarity, while guiding nurses to use the clock method, accurate edge descriptions, and wound bed % documentation (all required in best practice).

CHAPTER 14

The Four Phases of Wounds Healing

1. Hemostasis (Immediate – Minutes to Hours)

Purpose: Stop the bleeding and form the initial clot.

What Happens: Blood vessels constrict, platelets clump together, and clotting factors form a fibrin mesh.

Key Signs: Bleeding slows or stops, a clot forms at the wound site.

Goal: Create a temporary barrier to prevent further blood loss and protect against pathogens. This phase is essential for stabilizing the wound and creating the foundation for subsequent healing.

Hemostasis Phase

Immediate – Minutes to Hours

Purpose: Stop the bleeding and form the initial clot.

What happens: Blood vessels constrict, platelets clump together, and clotting factors form a fibrin meh.

Key signs: Bleeding slows or stops, clot forms at wound site

Goal: Create a temporary barrier to prevent further blood loss and protect against pathogens

Post-op Day 5 **After 2 Weeks**

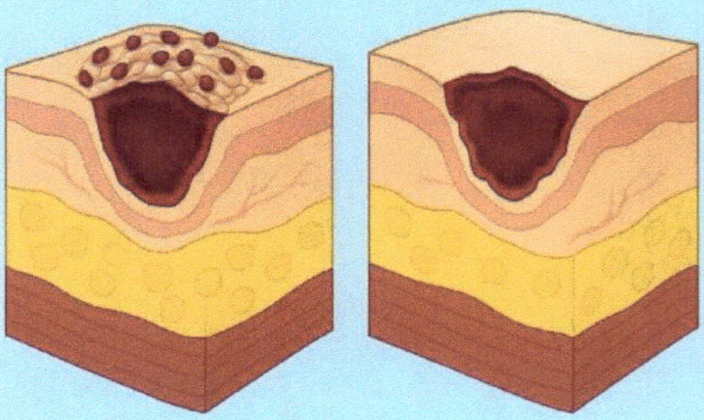

2. Inflammatory Phase (Hours to ~ 4 Days)

Purpose: Cleanse the wound of debris and bacteria.

What Happens: Blood vessels dilate, allowing white blood cells (especially neutrophils and macrophages) to enter the wound and remove bacteria and dead tissue.

Key Signs: Redness, warmth, swelling, and pain (normal in this phase).

Goal: Prevent infection and prepare wound bed for new tissue growth.

Inflammatory Phase
(Hours to ~4 Days)

Purpose:
Cleanse the wound of debris and bacteria.

What happens:
Blood vessels dilate, allowing white blood cells (especially neutrophils and macrophages) to enter the wound and remove bacteria and dead tissue.

Key signs:
Redness, warmth, swelling, and pain (normal in this phase)

Goal:
Prevent infection and prepare wound bed for new tissue growth

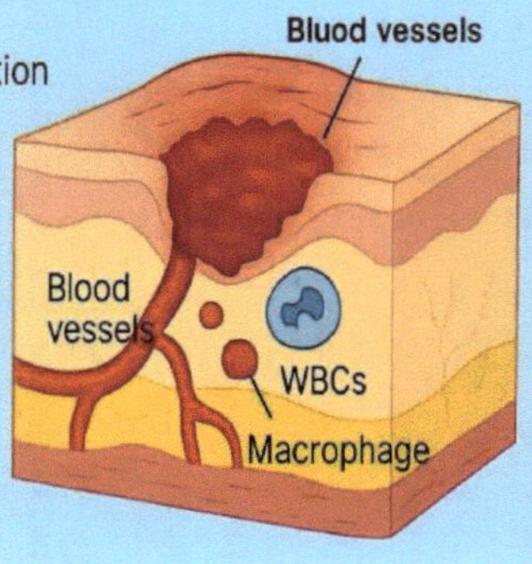

3. Proliferative Phase (4 Days to ~ 3 Weeks)

Purpose: Build new tissue and close the wound.

What Happens: Fibroblasts produce collagen, new blood vessels form (angiogenesis), and granulation tissue fills the wound. Epithelial cells migrate across the wound surface.

Key Signs: Pink/red moist tissue, decreased drainage, wound edges beginning to contract.

Goal: Replace lost tissue and restore the skin barrier.

3. Proliferative Phase
(4 Days to ~ 3 Weeks)

Purpose: Build new tissue and close the wound.

What happens: Fibroblasts produce collagen, new blood vessels form (angiogene-), and granulation tissue fills the wound. Epithelial cells migrate across the wound surface.

Key signs: Pink/red moist tissue, decreased drainage, wound edges beginning to contract

Goal: Replace lost tissue and restore skin barrier.

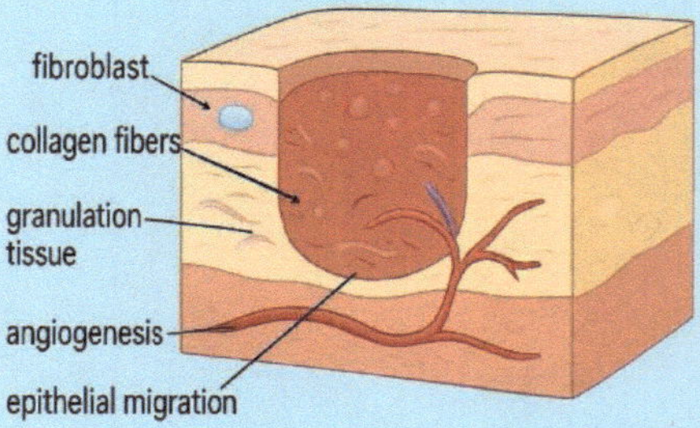

4. Maturation/Remodeling Phase (3 Weeks to Months or Years)

Purpose: Strengthen and reorganize tissue.

What Happens: Collagen fibers reorganize into stronger cross-linked patterns, scar tissue forms, and vascularity decreases. This remodeling continues for months and may last up to 2 years, depending on wound size and patient factors.

Key Signs: Scar becomes paler, thinner, and less vascular over time.

Goal: Restore tensile strength (scar tissue reaches about 80% of original skin strength).

Maturation / Remodeling Phase

(3 Weeks to Months or Years)

Purpose:
Strengthen and reorganize tissue.

What happens:
Collagen fibers reorganize into stronger cross-linked patterns, scar tissue forms, and vascularity decreases

Key signs:
Scar becomes paler, thinner, and less vascular over time

Goal:
Restore tensile strength (scar tissue reaches about 80% of original skin strength)

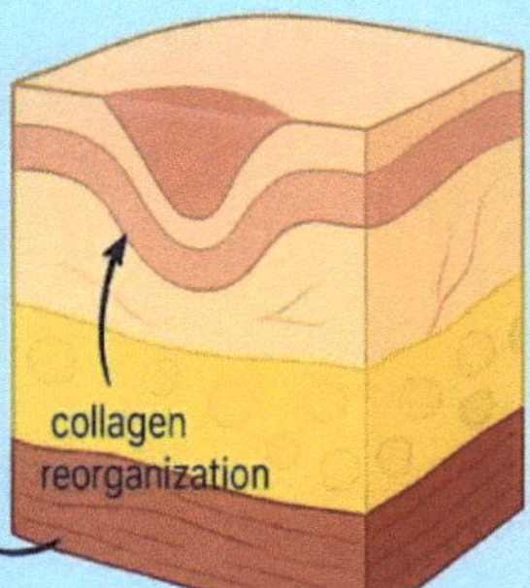

CHAPTER 15
Non-Healing Wounds

What to Do if a Wound Is Non-Healing

Definition of a Non-Healing Wound

A wound is considered non-healing when it fails to show measurable progress through the normal stages of healing (hemostasis, inflammation, proliferation, remodeling) within 4–6 weeks, despite standard wound care. Non-healing wounds are often chronic in nature and may be complicated by poor circulation, infection, or systemic health conditions.

Common examples: pressure injuries, diabetic ulcers, arterial or venous ulcers, post-surgical wounds.

Steps to Take if a Wound Is Non-Healing

1. Reassess the Patient Holistically

- **Medical status:** Check for comorbidities (diabetes, peripheral vascular disease, immunosuppression, renal/hepatic disease, cardiac failure, or thyroid disorders).
- **Nutrition:** Ensure adequate protein, vitamins (A, C, E), and minerals (zinc, iron).
- **Medications:** Steroids, chemotherapy, or anticoagulants can impair healing.

- **Blood sugar control:** Hyperglycemia significantly delays wound repair.
- **Lifestyle:** Assess for smoking, alcohol use, or sedentary behavior, as these directly impair healing.

2. Reevaluate the Wound

- Size, depth, tissue type, drainage, edges, peri-wound skin.
- Look for biofilm or infection (slough, foul odor, delayed granulation, or persistent pain).
- Assess for ischemia or poor blood flow using tools like Ankle-Brachial Index (ABI) or Doppler ultrasound.

3. Address Underlying Causes

- **Pressure Injuries:** Optimize offloading, repositioning, special mattresses/cushions.
- **Diabetic Wounds:** Strict glycemic control, offloading with specialized footwear, podiatry review, and regular foot inspections.
- **Arterial Ulcers:** Vascular consult, consider revascularization if severe ischemia, optimize blood pressure and lipid management.
- **Venous Ulcers:** Compression therapy to improve venous return, leg elevation, and exercise to support calf-muscle pump function.

4. Optimize Local Wound Care

- **Debridement:** Remove necrotic tissue and biofilm (sharp, enzymatic, autolytic, mechanical).

- **Moisture Balance:** Maintain a moist environment, but avoid maceration.
- **Dressing Choice:** Match to wound type and exudate (e.g., foam for heavy drainage, hydrocolloid for shallow wounds, alginate for bleeding wounds, hydrogels for dry necrotic wounds).
- **Infection Control:** Topical antimicrobials (silver dressings, iodine-based products) or systemic antibiotics if infection is systemic.
- **Pain Management:** Ensure adequate analgesia, as uncontrolled pain may limit adherence to care.

5. Advanced Therapies if Standard Care Fails

- **Negative Pressure Wound Therapy (NPWT):** Enhances granulation and fluid removal.
- **Growth Factors or Biologics:** e.g., platelet-derived growth factor, skin substitutes.
- **Hyperbaric Oxygen Therapy (HBOT):** Especially useful in diabetic foot ulcers and arterial ulcers.
- **Electrical Stimulation / Ultrasound Therapy:** Can stimulate healing.
- **Skin Grafts or Flap Surgery:** Consider in cases of large, non-healing wounds after optimization of underlying causes.

6. Multidisciplinary Approach

- Involve a Wound Care Specialist / WOCN.
- **Referrals:** A vascular surgeon, endocrinologist, podiatrist, infectious disease, or nutritionist, depending on wound type.

- **Psychological Support:** Chronic wounds often cause depression or anxiety. Referral to mental health professionals may improve overall outcomes.
- **Physiotherapy:** Encourage mobility where safe to improve circulation and general health.

7. Patient & Caregiver Education

- Daily skin inspection.
- Proper hygiene and dressing changes.
- Avoid smoking and alcohol (impairs circulation).
- Adherence to diet, medications, and offloading strategies.
- Teach early warning signs of infection (redness, swelling, new drainage).
- Encourage patient involvement in care, engagement improves healing adherence.

Summary

If A Wound Is Non-Healing:

- Step back and reassess the whole patient.
- Identify and treat underlying causes (pressure, poor circulation, infection, diabetes).
- Reevaluate wound management (debridement, dressing, infection control).
- Escalate to advanced therapies and specialists if no improvement.
- Empower the patient and caregivers through education and support, as long-term commitment is essential for healing.

Non-Healing Wound

A wound is considered non-healing when it fails to show measurable progress through the normal stages of healing (hemostasis, inflammation, proliferation, remodeling) within 4–6 weeks, despite standard care.

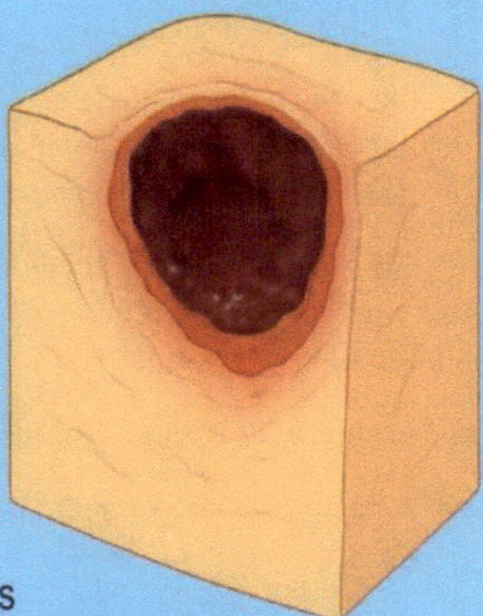

Common examples:

- Pressure injuries
- Diabetic ulcers
- Arterial ulcers
- Venous ulcers
- Post-surgical wounds

CHAPTER 16

When to Apply a Wound VAC

You should consider Negative Pressure Wound Therapy (NPWT) when the wound is not healing with standard care despite appropriate debridement, dressings, and infection control.

- Chronic wounds (pressure injuries, diabetic foot ulcers, venous/arterial ulcers) that show little to no progress after 2–4 weeks of conventional treatment.
- Large Tissue Loss
- Deep wounds, cavities, or wounds with tunneling/undermining.
- Wounds that require granulation tissue to fill in.
- Moderate to Heavy Drainage

VAC helps remove excess exudate and keep the wound environment balanced. Prevents maceration of peri-wound skin.

Post-Surgical with Risk of Complications

- Open abdominal wounds (laparotomy incisions left open).
- Orthopedic or trauma wounds with exposed bone, tendon, or hardware.
- Flaps and grafts – VAC improves perfusion and secures grafts in place.

- Reduces risk of surgical site infections by lowering bacterial load.

When a Clean, Granulating Bed Is Needed

- VAC promotes granulation tissue formation and wound contraction.
- Useful as a "bridge therapy" before surgical closure or skin grafting.
- Encourages faster epithelialization and may shorten overall healing time.

When NOT to Use Wound VAC (Contraindications)

You should avoid NPWT if the wound has:

- Necrotic tissue/eschar present → must debride first.
- Untreated osteomyelitis (bone infection).
- Exposed blood vessels, organs, or anastomotic sites without protective coverage.
- Malignant wound/tumor tissue in the wound bed.
- Uncontrolled bleeding or coagulopathy.
- Fragile skin or ischemic tissue without adequate perfusion.
- Allergy or hypersensitivity to dressing components (foam, drape, adhesives).
- Inadequate hemostasis immediately post-debridement.

Clinical Example

Appropriate Use: A diabetic foot ulcer with clean granulation tissue, heavy drainage, and deep undermining not healing after 3 weeks of moist dressings → Start VAC.

Not Appropriate Use: A heel ulcer covered in hard black eschar with poor pulses → First, revascularize and/or debride, then consider VAC.

Summary

Apply Wound VAC:

- On clean, debrided wounds with delayed healing, moderate/heavy drainage, or tissue loss.
- To promote granulation, decrease edema, and prepare for closure or grafting.
- As an adjunct to standard wound care, not a replacement for addressing underlying causes (infection, ischemia, diabetes).

Avoid if necrosis, untreated infection, exposed vessels/organs, or malignancy are present.

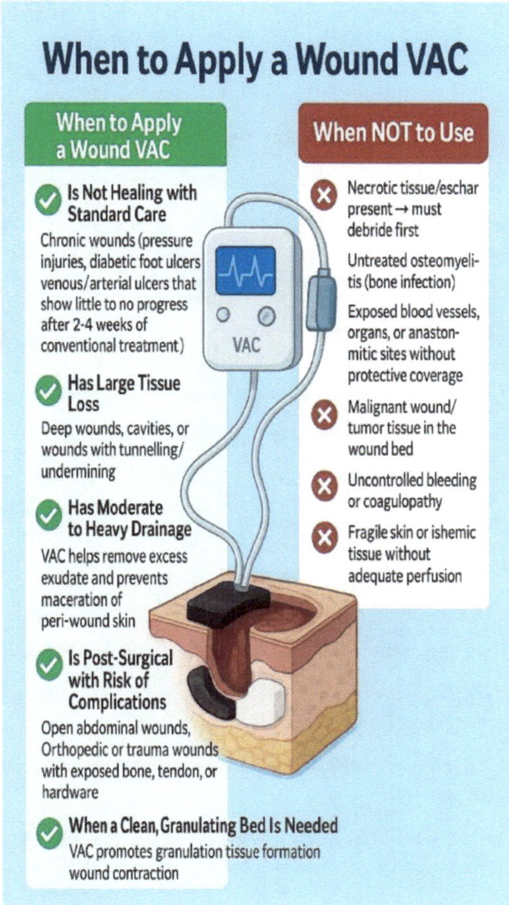
When to Apply a Wound VAC
When to Apply a Wound VAC
Is Not Healing with Standard Care
Chronic wounds (pressure injuries, diabetic foot ulcers venous/arterial ulcers that show little to no progress after 2-4 weeks of conventional treatment)
Has Large Tissue Loss
Deep wounds, cavities, or wounds with tunnelling/ undermining
Has Moderate to Heavy Drainage
VAC helps remove excess exudate and prevents maceration of peri-wound skin
Is Post-Surgical with Risk of Complications
Open abdominal wounds, Orthopedic or trauma wounds with exposed bone, tendon, or hardware
When a Clean, Granulating Bed Is Needed
VAC promotes granulation tissue formation wound contraction
VAC
When NOT to Use
Necrotic tissue/eschar present → must debride first
Untreated osteomyelitis (bone infection)
Exposed blood vessels, organs, or anastonmitic sites without protective coverage
Malignant wound/ tumor tissue in the wound bed
Uncontrolled bleeding or coagulopathy
Fragile skin or ishemic tissue without adequate perfusion

WOCN-Recommended Types of Wound Cleansers

1. Normal Saline (0.9% Sodium Chloride Solution)

Use: Standard for most acute and chronic wounds.

Benefits: Non-cytotoxic, isotonic, safe for all wound types.

Additional Notes: Readily available, inexpensive, and does not interfere with normal wound healing. Best used for daily cleansing and irrigation in wounds that do not require antimicrobial action.

2. Sterile Water

Use: For low-risk wounds or when saline is unavailable.

Benefits: Non-toxic, gentle on tissues.

Additional Notes: Lacks electrolytes, so not as physiologically balanced as saline. Still safe for superficial abrasions, minor cuts, and post-surgical wounds when infection risk is low.

3. Commercial Wound Cleansers (Surfactant-based)

Use: In wounds with biofilm, slough, or moderate debris.

Benefits: Contains mild surfactants that aid in removing debris, exudate, and biofilm.

Examples of Ingredients: Poloxamer, cocamidopropyl betaine, or other amphoteric agents.

Additional Notes: Many of these cleansers are packaged in spray or foam delivery systems to reduce trauma. They are especially helpful for chronic wounds (e.g., diabetic ulcers, venous leg ulcers) where biofilm may delay healing.

Antiseptic Wound Cleansers (Used Selectively Based on WOCN Guidelines)

1. Polyhexamethylene Biguanide (PHMB)

Use: For wounds with critical colonization or local infection.

Additional Notes: Broad-spectrum antimicrobial with low cytotoxicity. Can be used long-term in chronic wounds, especially pressure injuries.

2. Hypochlorous Acid Solutions

Use: Effective against pathogens, low cytotoxicity.

Additional Notes: Mimics natural neutrophil activity, making it safe for frequent use. Effective in reducing odor and biofilm without harming granulation tissue.

3. Superoxidized Solutions

Use: Antimicrobial properties, safe for delicate tissue.

Additional Notes: Effective against a wide range of bacteria, fungi, and viruses. Often used in wounds with high infection risk or compromised immune patients.

4. Povidone-Iodine, Dakin's Solution (Sodium Hypochlorite)

Caution: Used sparingly and short-term due to cytotoxicity.

Recommended For: Infected wounds with heavy bioburden.

Additional Notes: These solutions can delay epithelialization if overused. WOCN suggests using them in acute infection management or as a short "reset" before transitioning back to non-cytotoxic cleansers.

5. Acetic Acid Solution (0.25% - 1%)

Use: Effective against Pseudomonas aeruginosa infections.

Note: Use with caution to minimize tissue irritation.

Additional Notes: Best reserved for wounds with greenish-blue drainage suggestive of *Pseudomonas*. Therapy is usually short-term until cultures confirm bacterial reduction.

WOCN General Recommendations For Wound Cleansing

- Use room temperature or body-temperature solutions.
- Apply gentle pressure (4-15 psi) to avoid tissue trauma.
- Avoid cytotoxic agents (like hydrogen peroxide, iodine, or alcohol) unless absolutely indicated.
- Always cleanse before applying dressings, ensuring removal of old exudate and reducing bacterial load.
- Frequency of cleansing depends on wound condition: daily for heavily draining or contaminated wounds, less often for stable, dry wounds.

Tailor The Cleanser Choice Based On:

- Wound contamination level
- Presence of infection
- Tissue type exposed (granulation, slough, necrotic)

CHAPTER 17

The Future of Wound Care

Wound care has come a long way from basic gauze and antiseptic solutions. Advances in science, technology, and patient-centered care are shaping a future where wound healing is not only faster but also more personalized and precise. As healthcare continues to evolve, nurses and clinicians must prepare to integrate innovations that will redefine wound assessment, treatment, and prevention. This chapter explores emerging trends and the technologies that are transforming wound care into a discipline of precision medicine, innovation, and holistic care.

1. DIGITAL TECHNOLOGY & ARTIFICIAL INTELLIGENCE (AI)

I. Smart Imaging and Measurement

Traditional wound measurement using rulers and cotton swabs is being replaced by digital wound imaging systems. These devices use 3D cameras and AI algorithms to capture accurate wound dimensions, tissue composition, and healing progression. They reduce subjectivity in assessment and allow for precise tracking over time. Some systems even create a digital "wound twin" for longitudinal comparison, enabling clinicians to monitor microscopic changes invisible to the naked eye.

II. AI-Powered Decision Support

Artificial intelligence is increasingly being used to analyze wound data and recommend evidence-based treatment plans. AI-driven platforms can flag early signs of infection, suggest appropriate dressings, and predict healing times based on patient-specific factors such as comorbidities, nutrition, and vascular status. As datasets expand, AI will evolve into predictive engines that anticipate complications before they arise, shifting wound care from reactive to proactive practice.

III. Remote Monitoring & Telehealth

With the growth of home health, telehealth wound care is becoming standard practice. Patients and caregivers can upload wound photos through secure apps, allowing clinicians to evaluate healing remotely. This approach improves access, reduces hospital visits, and supports real-time intervention when complications arise. Future telehealth systems may include AI-driven chatbots, wearable sensors, and real-time video consultations, making continuous wound surveillance possible in nearly any setting.

2. SMART DRESSINGS & BIOMATERIALS

I. Sensor-Embedded Dressings

Researchers are developing smart bandages equipped with biosensors that monitor wound pH, oxygen levels, moisture, and bacterial load. These dressings can transmit data to healthcare providers, alerting them to infection or delayed healing before symptoms appear. This enables earlier intervention, reduces hospitalizations, and improves patient outcomes by promoting timely care.

II. Drug-Delivering Dressings

Future dressings may not only cover wounds but also release antibiotics, growth factors, or pain medications directly into the wound bed, providing targeted therapy and reducing systemic side effects. Personalized drug-delivery bandages may even be 3D-printed to match a patient's wound profile, ensuring therapy is highly specific and cost-effective.

III. Nanotechnology in Wound Care

Nanoparticles with antimicrobial properties are being incorporated into dressings to combat biofilm and resistant organisms. Nanofibers can also mimic the extracellular matrix, creating an ideal scaffold for tissue regeneration.

3. BIOLOGICS, REGENERATIVE MEDICINE & STEM CELLS

I. Growth Factor Therapies

Recombinant growth factors are being refined to stimulate angiogenesis (blood vessel formation), fibroblast proliferation, and collagen synthesis, accelerating healing in chronic wounds.

II. Stem Cell Applications

Stem cell therapy is one of the most promising frontiers in wound care. Stem cells harvested from bone marrow, adipose tissue, or cord blood can differentiate into skin cells, potentially regenerating tissue that would otherwise form chronic, non-healing wounds. Clinical trials are also exploring exosomes (tiny particles secreted by stem cells) that may deliver regenerative signals without the risks of direct stem cell transplantation.

III. Tissue Engineering & Skin Substitutes

Laboratories are developing bioengineered skin substitutes using 3D printing and tissue scaffolding. These products act as temporary or permanent coverings, promoting healing in burns, diabetic ulcers, and surgical wounds.

4. HYPERBARIC OXYGEN & ADVANCED THERAPIES

I. Hyperbaric Oxygen Therapy (HBOT)

While already in use for select wounds, HBOT continues to be studied and refined. Future innovations may make HBOT more portable and accessible for home health patients with chronic wounds. Emerging research is also exploring "nanobubble-based oxygen therapy," which could deliver oxygen directly into tissues through injectable solutions or topical applications.

II. Electrical & Ultrasound Stimulation

Emerging evidence supports the role of low-frequency ultrasound and electrical stimulation in accelerating healing by stimulating cellular activity and improving perfusion. Devices may become more compact, making them suitable for bedside or home use.

5. PRECISION & PERSONALIZED WOUND CARE

- The future of wound care will increasingly move toward personalized medicine:
- Genomics and proteomics may reveal why some individuals heal poorly.
- Tailored treatment plans will consider genetics, comorbidities, and microbiome composition.
- Predictive analytics will help determine which patients are at the highest risk for chronic wounds, enabling early preventive interventions.

6. GLOBAL ACCESSIBILITY & EQUITY IN WOUND CARE

As advanced technologies emerge, an equally important priority is ensuring equitable access. Many patients with chronic wounds live in resource-limited settings. Innovations must be adapted into cost-effective, scalable solutions that can be deployed in low- and middle-income countries. Nurses will play a key role in bridging this gap through education, advocacy, and community-based wound care models.

7. THE NURSE'S ROLE IN THE FUTURE OF WOUND CARE

- **Technology Adapters:** Nurses will need to integrate AI tools, digital imaging, and smart dressings into daily practice.

- **Educators & Advocates:** As patients gain access to new therapies, nurses must educate them on safe use and expectations.
- **Leaders in Prevention:** With prevention remaining the most cost-effective strategy, nurses will continue to lead in risk assessment, early detection, and patient education.
- **Interdisciplinary Collaborators:** Future wound care requires collaboration among nurses, physicians, nutritionists, mental health providers, and engineers developing wound technologies.

CONCLUSION

The future of wound care is moving toward integration of technology, biology, and holistic nursing care. From smart dressings that "think" to stem cell therapies that regenerate tissue, the next generation of wound care will be proactive, personalized, and precise. For nurses, this means staying at the forefront of education, embracing innovation, and always centering care on the patient's healing journey.

The message is clear: wound care is no longer just about closing a wound—it is about restoring health, dignity, and quality of life through cutting-edge science and compassionate care. By combining human touch with technological innovation, the future promises not only longer lives but also better lives for patients around the world.

CHAPTER 18
Conclusion

Wound care is not just about dressing a site of injury; it is about restoring dignity, preventing suffering, and enabling healing in its fullest sense. Throughout this guide, we have walked through the layers of evidence-based practice, practical techniques, and clinical wisdom that every nurse can apply at the bedside. The effectiveness of this book lies in its approach: it equips you to see beyond the surface of a wound, to interpret its story, and to respond with interventions that produce measurable, lasting results. Every chapter has been designed to connect theory with practice, bridging the gap between textbook knowledge and real-world clinical decision-making.

When wound care is approached systematically—through accurate assessment, timely intervention, vigilant monitoring, and patient-centered education—the outcomes are clear: wounds heal faster, complications are reduced, and quality of life is improved. This book provides not just knowledge, but a pathway for consistent excellence. It emphasizes prevention as strongly as treatment, recognizing that avoiding wounds altogether is as critical as managing those that occur. Each principle shared is designed to strengthen your confidence, sharpen your skills, and transform your practice into one that achieves better outcomes with fewer setbacks.

As you step forward, remember: every wound you encounter is an opportunity to apply science, skill, and compassion in equal measure. Healing is not a linear process, and setbacks are common, but the nurse's role is to remain steadfast, adaptable, and patient-focused. Let this guide be your companion in achieving the highest standards of care. By committing to continuous learning, disciplined technique, and holistic attention to the patient, you are positioned to make a profound difference. May your practice reflect the truth that effective wound care is not only possible—it is within your hands. With each patient encounter, you are not simply treating tissue; you are rebuilding trust, hope, and resilience.

GLOSSARY

Term	Definition
Alginate Dressing	Highly absorbent dressing derived from seaweed, used for wounds with heavy exudate.
Autolytic Debridement	Natural process of the body using moisture and enzymes to break down dead tissue.
Biofilm	A structured community of microorganisms enclosed in a protective layer, delaying wound healing.
Cellulitis	Infection of skin and soft tissues characterized by redness, warmth, swelling, and pain.
Debridement	Removal of non-viable tissue from a wound to promote healing (surgical, enzymatic, mechanical, autolytic).
Erythema	Redness of the skin, often a sign of inflammation or infection.
Fibrin	A protein involved in clot formation and wound healing.
Granulation Tissue	New connective tissue and tiny blood vessels that form on the wound surface during healing.

Term	Definition
Hypergranulation	Excessive granulation tissue that rises above the wound margins, delaying epithelialization.
Ischemia	Inadequate blood supply to tissue, often leading to ulceration or necrosis.
Keratinocytes	Skin cells responsible for re-epithelialization of a wound.
Maceration	Softening and breakdown of skin due to prolonged exposure to moisture.
Necrosis	Death of tissue, appearing black, brown, or grey; may be dry or moist.
Offloading	Redistributing pressure away from a wound site, especially in diabetic foot ulcers.
Pain (Wound-Related)	Pain directly caused by the wound, including nociceptive or neuropathic components.
Pressure Ulcer	Localized injury to the skin and/or underlying tissue, typically over a bony prominence, caused by pressure.
Slough	Yellow/white stringy tissue composed of dead cells and wound debris, often requiring debridement.
Tunneling	Channel extending from a wound into or through subcutaneous tissue or muscle.
Undermining	Erosion of tissue under wound edges, forming a pocket beneath intact skin.
Venous Insufficiency	Failure of veins to return blood efficiently, leading to edema and ulceration.

Term	Definition
Wound Bed	The base of the wound, including granulation tissue, slough, or necrotic tissue.

NOTES

NOTES

NOTES

NOTES

NOTES

NOTES

NOTES

NOTES

NOTES

NOTES

NOTES

NOTES

NOTES

NOTES

NOTES

REFERENCES

1. Baranoski, S., & Ayello, E. A. (2020). Wound care essentials: Practice principles (5th ed.). Wolters Kluwer.
2. Bryant, R. A., & Nix, D. P. (2016). Acute and chronic wounds: Current management concepts (5th ed.). Elsevier.
3. European Wound Management Association (EWMA). (2013). Debridement: An updated overview and clarification of the principle role of debridement. Journal of Wound Care, 22(Suppl 1), S1–S49. https://doi.org/10.12968/jowc.2013.22.Sup1.S1
4. National Pressure Injury Advisory Panel (NPIAP), European Pressure Ulcer Advisory Panel (EPUAP), & Pan Pacific Pressure Injury Alliance (PPPIA). (2019). Prevention and treatment of pressure ulcers/injuries: Clinical practice guideline. Emily Haesler (Ed.). Cambridge Media. https://npiap.com/page/Guidelines
5. Sussman, C., & Bates-Jensen, B. M. (2012). Wound care: A collaborative practice manual for health professionals (4th ed.). Lippincott Williams & Wilkins.
6. Wound, Ostomy and Continence Nurses Society (WOCN). (2016, updated 2021). Guideline for prevention and management of pressure injuries (stages I–IV). WOCN Society. https://www.wocn.org/clinical-guidelines/

7. Agency for Healthcare Research and Quality (AHRQ). (2014). Pressure ulcer treatment strategies: Comparative effectiveness review. AHRQ Publication No. 12-EHC148-EF. https://www.ahrq.gov/patient safety/settings/long-term-care/resource/pressure-injury/index.html

www.ingramcontent.com/pod-product-compliance
Lightning Source LLC
LaVergne TN
LVHW051128210926
848482LV00001B/19
* 9 7 9 8 3 4 9 5 8 2 9 2 9 *